Aids to Obstetric

D1189278

For Churchill Livingstone:

Publisher: Timothy Horne
Project Editor: Barbara Simmons
Copy Editor: Alison Bowers
Project Controller: Nancy Arnott
Design Direction: Erik Bigland
Indexer: Anne McCarthy

Aids to Obstetrics and Gynaecology For MRCOG

Gordon M. Stirrat MA MD FRCOG
Professor of Obstetrics and Gynaecology
University of Bristol

FOURTH EDITION

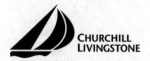

CHURCHILL LIVINGSTONE

NEW YORK EDINBURGH LONDON MADRID MELBOURNE SAN FRANCISCO
AND TOKYO 1997

CHURCHILL LIVINGSTONE
Medical Division of Pearson Professional Limited

Distributed in the United States of America by Churchill
Livingstone Inc., 650 Avenue of the Americas, New York, N.Y.
10011, and by associated companies, branches and
representatives throughout the world.
© Longman Group 1983
© Longman Group UK Limited 1987, 1991
© Pearson Professional Limited 1997

First edition 1981
Second edition 1987
Third edition 1991
Fourth edition first published 1997

ISBN 0 443 05535 1

British Library of Cataloguing in Publication Data
A catalogue record for this book is available from the British
Library.

Library of Congress Cataloging in Publication Data
A catalog record for this book is available from the Library of
Congress.

Medical knowledge is constantly changing. As information
becomes available, changes in treatment, procedures,
equipment and the use of drugs become necessary. The author
and publisher have, as far as it is possible, taken care to ensure
that the information given in the text is accurate and up-to-
date. However, readers are strongly advised to confirm that the
information, especially with regard to drug usage, complies
with current legislation and standards of practice.

The
publisher's
policy is to use
paper manufactured
from sustainable forests

Produced by the Publishing Technology Unit, Churchill
Livingstone
Printed in Singapore

Preface

The fundamental aim of this fourth edition is the same as those that have preceded it. That is to provide an authoritative, comprehensive guide to the essentials of obstetrics and gynaecology. Progress in knowledge and practice has resulted in an extensive revision of the content and style. In this I have, yet again, been considerably assisted by my friends and colleagues Simon Jackson, John Murdoch, Peter Soothill and Peter Wardle.

I have continued to depend on the work of a multitude of eminent authors, and the legacy of a series of outstanding teachers is gratefully acknowledged. The impact of 'Effective Care in Pregnancy and Childbirth' and the Cochrane Database of Pregnancy and Childbirth, to which frequent reference has been made in the text, cannot be overstated. There is, therefore, even greater reference to, and critical analysis of, 'evidence-based medicine' in this edition than before.

As usual, I have learned a great deal from preparing this edition. What has been written is up-to-date and as accurate as possible but, inevitably, with the passage of even a few years, new knowledge will supersede some of it. The reader should, therefore, approach the text with a properly critical attitude.

Teaching others continues to be a great joy and I remain grateful to Churchill Livingstone for, once more, giving me the opportunity to do so through my writing.

Bristol, 1997   G.M.S.

Contents

SECTION ONE
Obstetric care

1. Obstetric care

Obstetric care has four phases:
- pre-conception (p. 5)
- antenatal (p. 5)
- intrapartum (p. 129)
- postnatal (p. 171).

Its objectives are:
- *risk assessment*—to assess risk of harm to mother and baby
- *counselling*—to advise on the nature and extent of any perceived risks, and how to minimise or eradicate them
- *education*—to provide information on normal pregnancy and childbirth and give some guidance about pregnancy problems and possible interventions
- *treatment*—to treat any condition which might affect, or be affected by, the pregnancy
- *satisfaction*—to make the pregnancy and delivery as fulfilling yet as safe as possible.

RISK AND PREGNANCY

Risk is the probability that a particular event will occur.
- An 'at risk' pregnancy is one in which the probability of an adverse outcome in the mother and/or baby is greater than that for pregnant women in general.
- Factors associated with risk of a particular event are 'risk markers'.
- For the terms 'high risk' and 'low risk' to be useful, the probability, nature and extent of specific risks must be considered.
  —A high risk of one particular outcome does not necessarily imply a high risk of other adverse outcomes.
  —A low risk of a serious condition with a bad outcome should be given more weight than a high risk of a lesser problem which has minor effects.
  —Perception of risk varies among individuals.
- A guide to the extent of particular risks in pregnancy (e.g. pre-term birth, intrauterine growth retardation, congenital malformation or perinatal death) can be obtained from:
  —history and examination for presence of risk markers

—screening tests offered to all pregnant women (see p. 38)
—diagnostic tests for those in whom a screening test is positive, or who have clinical signs and symptoms.
- For a screening test to be of value it must:
  —predict the great majority of those who have the condition (*high positive predictive power*)
  —exclude those who do not have the condition (*high negative predictive power*).
- All screening tests have some *false-positive and false-negative* results.
  —The clinical value depends on the balance between them and the severity of the condition.
  —A test of value when the incidence of a condition is high will be of poorer predictive value in another population with a low incidence of the same condition.

Interventions
- Diagnostic and therapeutic interventions have their own intrinsic risk.
- On some occasions an intervention may cause the harm one is trying to prevent.
- An intervention without proven benefit cannot be justified on the basis that it will 'do no harm'.

RISK MARKERS ASSOCIATED WITH RISK OF ADVERSE OUTCOME TO BABY AND/OR MOTHER

The nature and extent of the risks are discussed in the text.

Physical factors
- Height <1.54 m
- Obesity—body mass index (BMI) >30/m²

Social factors
- Teenage pregnancy
- Maternal age >35 increasing further from 38 then 40 years
- High parity and low inter-pregnancy interval
- Poor socioeconomic conditions
- Alcohol intake >80 g/day
- Substance abuse

Genetic factors
- Family history of diabetes in first-degree relative
- Family or personal history of inheritable diseases, e.g. haemoglobinopathy, thrombophilia, etc.
- Congenital malformations in mother, family or previous child.

Obstetric/gynaecological factors

- History of subfertility or recurrent miscarriage
- Previous gynae. surgery, e.g. myomectomy, cone biopsy, pelvic floor repair
- Presence of sizeable fibroids
- Previous pre-term delivery or low birthweight infant
- Previous baby >4 kg
- Previous placental abruption or third-stage abnormality
- Previous caesarean section
- Previous stillbirth or neonatal death
- Previous third degree tear
- Elevated serum α-fetoprotein (AFP) levels in absence of NTD
- Multiple pregnancy

PRE-CONCEPTION CARE

It is important that care begins before pregnancy because:
- many women enter pregnancy poorly nourished, smoking heavily, and in a less than optimal state of health
- the most critical phase of fetal development is complete by the time of the first antenatal clinic attendance, and adverse factors have already begun to produce their effects.

Pre-conception clinics allow:
- women with chronic disease (e.g. diabetes) to become pregnant in as healthy a condition as possible
- dietary advice to be offered to those above or below ideal body weight
- encouragement to give up smoking and reduce alcohol ingestion
- advice to be given to those who are anxious, have had problems in a previous pregnancy, or who have a personal or family history of a congenitally malformed child
- rubella immunisation to be offered if the woman is susceptible
- baseline measures of weight and blood pressure to be obtained.

Much of this care is the proper responsibility of the primary health care team; however, obstetricians, physicians and clinical geneticists should be prepared to provide the benefit of their expertise.

ANTENATAL CARE

- Antenatal care is a screening system which aims to assess and obviate risk of harm to mother and baby.
- Traditional patterns of care were established over 50 years ago; their primary objective was to reduce maternal mortality and morbidity.

- Few of the measures used routinely today are of proven benefit.
- 'Proof' is not easy, given the difficulty in determining what outcomes should be measured, let alone measuring them!

BOOKING CLINIC

- Assessment of risk begins when the woman is seen by her midwife or general practitioner early in pregnancy (best within the first 8 weeks).
- The first hospital booking visit should take place around 12 and not later than 16 weeks' gestation.

ROUTINE BOOKING ASSESSMENT

- Administrative details, including age, marital status and gravidity, are recorded.
- An accurate menstrual history is important to assess gestational age.

History
- Medical and surgical; obstetric; family; social, smoking, alcohol and drug ingestion; inoculation risk (see p. 112).

Examination
- Weight; height; blood pressure; urinalysis for protein, blood and glucose
- General—chest, heart, breasts, etc.
- Abdominal—fundal height (if palpable), presence of any abnormal masses or tenderness
- Pelvic—routine vaginal examination is unnecessary
- Cervical smear if none within past 5 years
- Ultrasound scan (see p. 8).

Investigations
- FBC and check for haemoglobinopathy when indicated (see p. 43); ABO and Rh group and check for antibodies; rubella immunity; VDRL
- Biochemical screening for Down's syndrome (see p. 38) at 15 weeks (optional); hepatitis B status; HIV status in women at high risk (see p. 110) with their consent
- Screen for toxoplasmosis if at high risk (see p. 114)
- Mid-stream urine (MSU) for culture and sensitivity
- Chest X-ray (if at high risk of tuberculosis).

The appropriate pattern of antenatal care and place of delivery is determined based on maternal choice and the presence of risk markers (see above).

The policy must be continually re-appraised during pregnancy. Women at low risk of pregnancy problems can be delivered by their own midwife and GP.

Among the criteria for booking in a GP unit isolated from a maternity hospital or for home confinement are:
- second, third or fourth pregnancy under 35 years of age
- no medical, psychological or obstetric contraindications
- no recognised fetal risk (e.g. growth retardation; rhesus or other antibodies).

Individual cases can be discussed with the mother by the midwife, the GP, and the hospital team.

CONTINUING ANTENATAL CARE

The traditional pattern of care involved the woman being seen by a midwife and/or doctor every 4 weeks up to 28 weeks; every 2 weeks from 28 to 36 weeks, and weekly thereafter. This has not been proven to be necessary in women at low risk of developing complications, for whom the following schedule is suggested, shared between GP and hospital:

8–12 weeks	to GP to arrange booking and confirm dates
12–15 weeks	to consultant, hospital or peripheral clinic for booking, serology and screening tests (e.g. ultrasound, serum AFP)
26–28 weeks	to check fetal growth
36 weeks	to check presentation
40 weeks	pre-delivery assessment
41 weeks	to hospital if not delivered.

36 weeks, 40 weeks } with GP/midwife

Any additional visits should have a clearly specified objective, e.g. risk markers now present.

ROUTINE ASSESSMENTS

Every subsequent visit:
- urinalysis
- blood pressure
- exclude peripheral oedema
- measure and record fundal height (in centimetres above symphysis pubis).

Every visit in third trimester:
- fetal lie and presentation
- presence of fetal heart
- record patient awareness of fetal movement.

At 26 and 36 weeks (as a minimum):
- full blood count
- Rh-D antibodies in Rh-negative women and other antibodies if necessary.

The presence (or development) of adverse features demands closer attention than above and the introduction of more sophisticated methods of assessment of maternal and fetal welfare (see pp. 57–60). Among the risk markers which can arise during pregnancy are:

- vaginal bleeding
- hypertension
- proteinuria
- persistent glycosuria
- urinary tract or other infections
- oligohydramnios
- polyhydramnios
- marked reduction in fetal movements in last trimester
- intrauterine growth retardation (p. 60).
- malpresentations (after 34 weeks).

ULTRASOUND IN ANTENATAL CARE

Among the clinical situations in which ultrasonic imaging is most useful are:

- assessment of vaginal bleeding and/or abdominal pain in early pregnancy. This can be done most efficiently and effectively within an organised early pregnancy problem clinic (see p. 17)
- accurate ascertainment of gestational age—menstrual history can be unreliable in up to 45% of women
- allowing more exact interpretation of serum AFP levels
- exclusion of multiple pregnancy
- examination of the fetus for severe congenital anomaly as part of a screening programme (see below) or when the individual risk is high; and before amniocentesis or chorionic villus sampling
- to check fetal size and liquor volume when the uterus is small or large for dates
- monitoring fetal growth in high-risk pregnancies (see p. 54). The addition of Doppler ultrasound assessment of fetal umbilical artery waveforms can be useful in this circumstance *but not as a routine in low-risk pregnancies*
- ascertaining the placental site and identifying the source of some antepartum haemorrhages (APH)
- determination of fetal presentation if it is unclear by palpation
- discovering fetal attitude in malpresentations
- more confident timing of any obstetric intervention (e.g. for postmaturity).

ROUTINE ULTRASOUND SCANS?

- Although a policy of routine scanning has not been shown significantly to affect pregnancy outcome, it is generally considered to be of clinical value.
- *Each centre must have a clear policy.*

- If ultrasound scanning is offered the suggested optimal programme is:
  - *A first scan at around 12 weeks' gestation* can confirm continuing pregnancy and gestational age (allows better counselling for, and accurate timing of, Down's screening tests at 15 weeks); and exclude such major anomalies as anencephaly (allows safer termination of pregnancy)
  - *A second scan at 20 weeks* has the best predictive value in the detection of serious malformations (earlier scanning is more likely to miss serious cardiac anomalies)
  - No further scanning is indicated in the absence of any risk markers
  - Scans must be performed (or supervised) only by fully trained personnel (see below).

SAFETY OF ULTRASOUND

- There is no good evidence that ultrasound is anything but safe for mother, baby and operator (see Further Reading).
- *The skill of the operator is of prime importance. Misleading information will lead to wrong management decisions.*

OTHER ASPECTS OF CARE

This is an important time to provide health education and advice on, for example, diet, dental care, smoking (avoid it), coitus (no association with adverse pregnancy outcome), substance abuse and maternity benefits.

Preparation for labour and breast-feeding should begin well in advance.

FURTHER READING

Berryman J, Thorpe K, Windridge K 1995 Older mothers—conception, pregnancy and birth after 35. Pandora, London

Chamberlain G (ed) 1995 Turnbull's obstetrics. Churchill Livingstone, Edinburgh

The Cochrane Collaboration 1995 Cochrane Pregnancy and Childbirth Database. BMJ Publishing Group, London

Enkin M, Kierse M J N C, Chalmers I (eds) 1989 Effective care in pregnancy and childbirth. Vol.1: Pregnancy. Oxford University Press, Oxford

James D K, Stirrat G M 1988 Pregnancy and risk. Wiley, Chichester

James D K, Steer P J, Weiner C P, Gonik B (eds) 1994 High risk pregnancy—management options. Saunders, London

Pearson V 1994 Preconception care. Health Care Evaluation Unit, University of Bristol, Bristol

Pearson V 1994 Antenatal ultrasound screening. Health Care Evaluation Unit, University of Bristol, Bristol

Pearson V 1994 Frequency and timing of antenatal visits. Health Care Evaluation Unit, University of Bristol, Bristol

RCOG 1990 Report of Working Party on routine ultrasound examination in pregnancy. RCOG, London

RCOG 1995 Report of Joint Working Group on Organisational Standards for Maternity Services. RCOG, London

2. Pregnancy physiology

Male and female fertility is discussed on pages 202–205.
  The timing of some crucial events in early pregnancy is shown in Table 2.1.

Table 2.1

Event	Time from fertilisation
First cleavage	30 hours
Second cleavage	40 hours
Morula formed (16-cell stage to formation of blastocyst)	50 to 60 hours
Morula reaches uterus and blastocyst forms (from 50- to 60-cell stage)	4 to 5 days
Implantation begins	7 days
Implantation is complete	14 days
Primary, secondary then tertiary villi form sequentially	12 to 16 days
Fetal circulation becomes established	21 to 28 days

MATERNAL ADAPTATION TO PREGNANCY

- This involves fundamental physiological changes in *every* system in the body.
- These changes *must* occur if pregnancy is to progress normally.
- Many pregnancy complications (even those which only become apparent in the third trimester) are determined because physiological adaptation does not occur.
- *Probably the most important single adaptation is to the vascular endothelium of the whole body.* This is particularly important in the placental bed.
- Most of these changes occur in the first 12 weeks of pregnancy.

SYSTEM OF COMMUNICATION BETWEEN MOTHER AND FETUS

The adaptation depends on signals passing between the embryo/fetus and the mother. Most of the signals emanate from the trophoblast mediated by, for example:

- cell-adhesion molecules (many of which act as growth factors or their receptors) and cytokines. These act locally on the decidua
- a large number of hormones for local and distant effects (e.g. oestrogens, progesterone, human chorionic gonadotrophin (hCG)).

PHYSIOLOGICAL CHANGES IN PREGNANCY

Haemodynamic changes in pregnancy

See Figure 2.1 for detail.

Cardiac output (CO) increases by up to 40% by 20 weeks and remains at that level thereafter.

Vascular resistance (VR) falls markedly due mainly to an increase in endothelial:

- vasodilatory prostacyclin (PGI$_2$) relative to vasoconstrictive thromboxane A$_2$ (TXA$_2$)
- nitric oxide (NO) which is a potent vasodilator and inhibitor of platelet activation
- inducible NO synthase (iNOS) is produced by the placenta, which may be a mechanism for controlling feto-placental perfusion pressure.

One of the systemic effects is that blood pressure (CO x VR) tends to fall—see Figure 2.2.

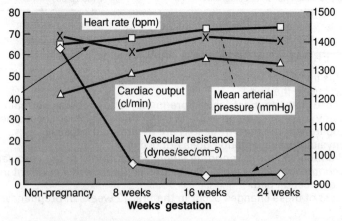

Fig 2.1   Haemodynamic changes in pregnancy

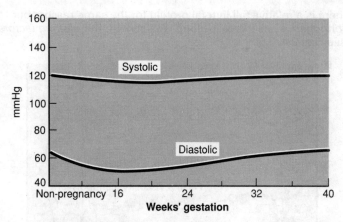

Fig 2.2 Blood pressure in pregnancy (supine)

Haematological system
See Figure 2.3 for detail.
- *Plasma volume* increases by up to 40%. Haematocrit tends to fall, because although there is an increase in red cell mass, it is relatively less than that of plasma volume.

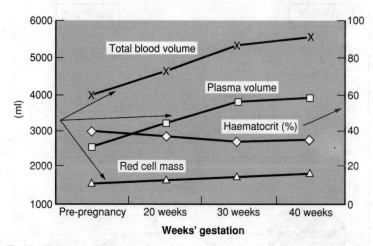

Fig 2.3 Haematological indices in pregnancy

- There is a relative fall in total protein for the same reason, but *fibrinogen* levels increase along with some other *clotting factors* (see Figs 2.4, 2.5).

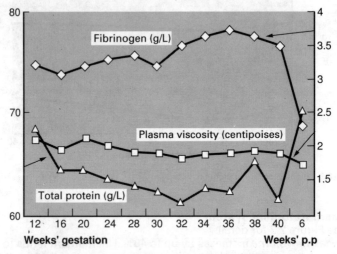

Fig 2.4 Levels in pregnancy of fibrinogen, plasma viscosity and total protein

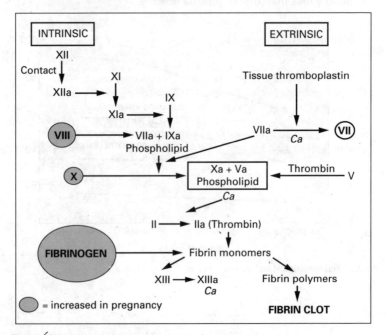

Fig 2.5 Blood coagulation system: changes in pregnancy

- This increased coagulability is further enhanced by the increase in *plasminogen inhibitors* (see Fig. 2.6).

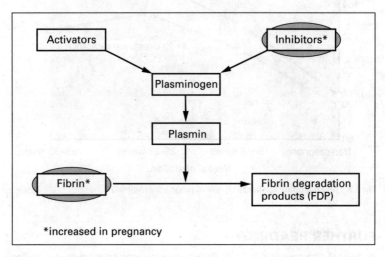

*increased in pregnancy

Fig 2.6   Fibrinolytic system: changes in pregnancy

Urinary system and water balance
- The *renal tracts* begin to dilate by 10 weeks of pregnancy (right > left). Dilatation persists for 12–16 weeks after delivery.
- *Renal blood flow* rises by about 75% in pregnancy with a resulting increase in *glomerular filtration rate* (GFR) as shown by increased inulin and creatinine clearance (see Fig. 2.7).
- *Total body water* increases by 6–8 L and *plasma osmolality* falls. The passage of normal urine volumes in the face of these is unique to pregnancy. It is due to a resetting of the osmoreceptors and the maintenance of arginine vasopressin (AVP) secretion.
- The pregnant woman expends considerable amounts of energy retaining sodium in face of these changes in body water.

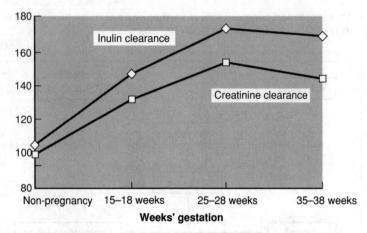

Fig 2.7   Mean glomerular filtration rate in pregnancy (ml/min)

FURTHER READING

de Swiet M, Chamberlain G V P 1992 Basic science in obstetrics and gynaecology, 2nd edn. Churchill Livingstone, Edinburgh
Hytten F, Chamberlain G V P (eds) 1990 Clinical physiology in obstetrics, 2nd edn. Blackwell Scientific, Oxford
Johnson M, Everitt B 1995 Essential reproduction, 4th edn. Blackwell Scientific, Oxford

3. Problems in early pregnancy

EARLY PREGNANCY PROBLEM CLINIC

Problems in early pregnancy, and some other gynaecological emergencies, are best dealt with in a specific clinic, the main elements of which are:
- direct daily access by GPs
- staffed by nurses, medical staff and radiographers trained in transvaginal ultrasound
- same day β-hCG testing available
- immediate admission possible when necessary with access to theatre during working hours.

ABORTION

Definition
- Biological—the expulsion or extraction of products of conception before fetal viability is achieved.
- Epidemiological (WHO)—the expulsion or extraction from its mother of an embryo or fetus weighing 500 g or less.
- Any fetus delivered and 'showing signs of life' becomes a potential livebirth and should be registered as such (see p. 165).

Ultrasound scan for diagnosis
- Each unit should have a written management policy to minimise the chances of evacuation of a live embryo in error.
- Two transvaginal scans at least 7 days apart are required before the death of an embryo can be confirmed.
- Only those adequately trained and experienced in ultrasound should carry out the examinations.
- The following features need to be recorded:
  - number of sacs
  - mean gestation sac diameter
  - presence of any haematoma
  - presence of a yolk sac
  - presence of an embryo
  - crown–rump length (CRL)
  - presence or absence of heart beat
  - appearance of ovaries
  - findings suggestive of ectopic pregnancy: tubal mass or fluid in pouch of Douglas.

SPONTANEOUS ABORTION (MISCARRIAGE)

Incidence
The loss rate among clinically recognised pregnancies is about 15%. It may rise to 50% if unrecognised pregnancies are included. Most occur within the first 14 weeks.

Potential causes
- No demonstrable cause—this is the commonest situation
- Chromosome anomalies may cause up to 25% of all miscarriages, particularly trisomy, XO and triploidy
- Anembryonic pregnancy ('blighted ovum'), abnormality of placental development
- Multiple pregnancy
- Uterine—e.g. congenital or acquired cervical incompetence; congenital uterine anomalies (classically occur in mid-trimester)
- Corpus luteum failure—it is more likely that the corpus luteum is failing because abortion is occurring rather than the converse; an increased miscarriage rate among women with polycystic ovary disease may relate to corpus luteum failure (see p. 188)
- Infections, e.g. rubella, cytomegalovirus, any acute pyrexial illness or condition causing peritonitis.

THREATENED ABORTION

The features are:
- amenorrhoea followed by slight vaginal bleeding
- no pain
- the uterus is the correct size for dates
- the cervix is closed.

If an ultrasonic scan can demonstrate a fetal heart there is a 90% chance that the pregnancy will progress satisfactorily. Bed rest is of no therapeutic value, and treatment with progestogens or hCG cannot be justified.

INEVITABLE (INCOMPLETE) ABORTION

The features are:
- amenorrhoea followed by heavy vaginal bleeding
- pain follows bleeding (cf. ectopic pregnancy)
- the uterus may be small, large or correct size for dates
- the cervix is dilating and products of conception may be passing through the os.

Management
- Up to 80% of women with an inevitable abortion will have no ultrasound scan evidence of retained products within 3 days of onset of signs and symptoms.

- Conservative management may be justified if:
  —gestation <13 weeks
  —hCG >50 but less than 1000 IU/L
  —transvaginal scan shows gestation sac diameter >15 mm but
    <50 mm.
- Active management is required if bleeding is heavy or the above
  are not fulfilled.
  —Give ergometrine 0.5 mg i.m. and arrange evacuation of the
    uterus.
  —If the uterus is larger than 12 weeks' size set up syntocinon
    infusion to cause reduction in uterine size before undertaking
    evacuation.
- The place of synthetic prostaglandin analogues (e.g. misoprostol
  400 µg) for 'medical evacuation' requires further evaluation.

COMPLETE ABORTION

The features are:
- amenorrhoea followed by a variable amount of bleeding which
  has now stopped
- the uterus is smaller than expected
- the cervix is closed.

Conservative management is indicated if the uterine cavity is
empty on transvaginal ultrasonic scan. If retained products are
suspected, manage as for inevitable miscarriage.

ANEMBRYONIC PREGNANCY ('BLIGHTED OVUM')

- A gestation sac develops in the absence of an embryo.
- The diagnosis is made if two transvaginal scans at least 7 days
  apart show a gestation sac of mean diameter >20 mm with no
  evidence of an embryo or yolk sac.
- Management—as for missed abortion.

MISSED ABORTION

Retention of the products of conception after death of the embryo
or fetus. The features are:
- amenorrhoea during which an episode of slight vaginal bleeding
  may or may not have occurred
- regression of earlier signs and symptoms of pregnancy
- uterus small-for-dates
- cervix is closed
- two transvaginal scans at least 7 days apart show an embryo
  with a crown–rump length >6 mm with no heart beat
- if the mean diameter of the gestation sac is <15 mm or the CRL
  is <6 mm repeat the examination in 2 weeks.

If left alone, resorption or spontaneous expulsion will occur but it is best to proceed to active management in most cases once a firm diagnosis has been made.

Active management

Option 1 If <9 weeks' gestation a combination of oral mifepristone followed by vaginal prostaglandin may be used. Contraindications to the use of prostaglandins include a history of asthma, cardiovascular disease and renal or hepatic failure.

Option 2 Uterus at or less than 12 weeks' size—proceed to careful aspiration of uterus under general anaesthesia (GA).

Option 3 Uterus greater than 12 weeks' size—use vaginal or extra-amniotic prostaglandins to induce abortion. Subsequent evacuation may be necessary.

SEPTIC ABORTION

- An incomplete abortion complicated by infection of the uterine contents. This may be due to criminal interference.
- The features are as for incomplete abortion accompanied by pyrexia (≥38°C) and tachycardia, general malaise, abdominal pain, marked pelvic tenderness and purulent vaginal loss.
- Other causes of an 'acute abdomen' and generalised infection must be excluded.

Pathogenesis
- The commonest infection organisms are *E. coli* (and other Gram-negative bacteria), streptococci (haemolytic and anaerobic), other anaerobes (e.g. *Bacteroides*) and *Staphylococcus*.
- Although infections with *Cl. perfringens* and *Cl. tetani* are infrequent now they are potentially lethal if not treated promptly and adequately.

Pathology
- The infection is usually mild (80%), being confined to the decidua but it can spread to the myometrium and beyond (15%).
- In the remainder (5%) more generalised signs and symptoms appear due to the release of endotoxins (see below).
- Endotoxic shock and disseminated intravascular coagulation may develop in these severe cases.

Investigation
- Take *cervical* (not vaginal) swabs for bacteriology in all cases and blood cultures if the pyrexia is at or greater than 38.4°C.
- In severe infections monitor fluid and electrolyte balance and check coagulation status.

Management
- Antibiotic therapy—for mild cases give a broad-spectrum antibiotic and metronidazole orally while awaiting the results of bacteriology cultures.
- In moderate and severe cases the intravenous route is preferred but metronidazole can be given rectally.
- Evacuation of the uterus—this is probably better deferred until reasonable tissue levels of antibiotics have been achieved (i.e. about 12 hours). The timing of intervention may of course be dictated by other circumstances.

RECURRENT MISCARRIAGE

Definition
Three or more consecutive miscarriages.
- Primary recurrent miscarriage—all pregnancies have ended in loss
- Secondary recurrent miscarriage—one (usually the first) pregnancy has proceeded to viability with all others ending in loss.

Incidence
Less than 1% of women of reproductive age.

Clinical management of recurrent miscarriage

Table 3.1   Clinical management of recurrent miscarriage

Associated factor	Investigation and diagnosis	Treatment	Comment
Anatomical disorders			
Uterine abnormalities	Hysterosalpingogram (HSG) or vaginal ultrasound	A septum can be divided by utriculoplasty or vaginally using an operating hysteroscope	Abdominal operation can cause infertility
Fibroids	Hysterosalpingogram (HSG) or vaginal ultrasound	Myomectomy	True role of fibroids unclear
Asherman's syndrome (intrauterine synechiae)	Hysteroscopy	Division of synechiae	Usually caused by multiple curettage
Cervical incompetence, congenital or acquired	HSG or vaginal ultrasound	Cervical cerclage	True diagnosis difficult and benefit from treatment uncertain

Problems in early pregnancy

Table 3.1   Clinical management of recurrent miscarriage (cont'd)

Associated factor	Investigation and diagnosis	Treatment	Comment
Genetic disorders			
Recurrent aneuploidy	Fetal karyotyping	None—occurs as a chance event or related to maternal age	Sporadic genetic disorders recurring consecutively by chance may explain many recurrent miscarriages
Parental balanced translocation	Parental karyotypes	Genetic counselling (see p. 48)	Accounts for 4% of cases
Molecular mutations	DNA analysis may be available in the future		Speculative
Endocrine factors			
Inadequate luteal phase	Luteal phase <10 days; progesterone levels <15 nmol/L in five consecutive cycles; endometrial biopsy(?)	Clomiphene, progesterone or hCG (empirical treatment not justified)	Reported incidence varies between 3 and 60%
Polycystic ovary disease associated with increased luteinising hormone (LH)	See p. 188	See p. 190	Role in recurrent losses becoming clearer
Thyroid function	Not justified	Not justified	Not a cause
Diabetes	Not justified	Not justified	Not a cause

Reproductive tract infections
Few data exist to support infection as a cause of recurrent pregnancy loss. Well-designed studies are necessary.

Table 3.1 Clinical management of recurrent miscarriage (cont'd)

Associated factor	Investigation and diagnosis	Treatment	Comment
Immunological causes			
Anti-cardiolipin (ACA) syndrome	Check APTT* routinely in all cases; carry out more detailed auto-immune screen and check specifically for anti-cardiolipin antibodies and lupus inhibitor if indicated (see p. 100)	Low-dose aspirin and/or steroids for women with ACA syndrome (see p. 100); *not* justified empirically	Tends to be associated with secondary recurrent miscarriage
Disorders of materno-fetal immune status	None routinely	The benefit of immuno-therapy is not proven	Scientific basis for investigation and therapy not strong
Psychological causes	?	'Tender loving care'	Evidence for this is no better and no worse than for several other 'causes'

*APTT: activated partial thromboplastin time

- Even after three consecutive losses the spontaneous chance of a successful pregnancy is over 60%.
- The success of all 'treatments' needs to be viewed with the spontaneous success rate in mind.
- When the women with a history of repeated miscarriages becomes pregnant she requires careful antenatal supervision. Poor reproductive performance tends also to be reflected in an increased incidence of other pregnancy complications.

FURTHER READING

Bennett M J, Edmonds D K 1987 Spontaneous and recurrent abortion. Blackwell Scientific, Oxford
Chamberlain G (ed) 1995 Turnbull's obstetrics. Churchill Livingstone, Edinburgh
Glasier A 1993 Drugs in Focus: 9 Mifepristone. Prescribers' Journal 33:156–161
James D K, Steer P J, Weiner C P, Gonik B (eds) 1994 High risk pregnancy—management options. Saunders, London

ECTOPIC PREGNANCY

Definition
The implantation of a pregnancy outside the uterine cavity.

Incidence
- The estimated incidence in England and Wales has risen from 12/1000 pregnancies in 1973–75 to 24/1000 in 1988–90.
- Women in age range 25–34 years comprise 65% of ectopics.
- After one ectopic the risk of recurrence is between 10 and 20%.

Maternal risk
- Ectopic pregnancy caused over 10% of all maternal deaths in 1988–90 and was the commonest cause of first-trimester deaths.
- The risk of death was about 2/1000 ectopics.
- 'Substandard care' contributed to almost 50% of the deaths.

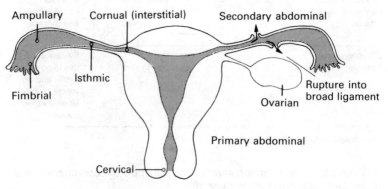

Fig 3.1   Sites of ectopic pregnancies

TUBAL PREGNANCY (95%)

Risk factors include:
- a history of infertility
- pelvic inflammatory disease
- pelvic operations (particularly tubal surgery)
- previous tubal pregnancy
- assisted conception (particularly IVF if tubes are patent and damaged)
- presence of an intrauterine device

There has also been a tendency to postpone pregnancy to the age range of greatest risk.

   Antibodies to *Chlamydia trachomatis* can be found in up to 80% and to *N. gonococcus* in up to 30% of women with ectopic pregnancy (compared with 40 and 4% respectively for intrauterine pregnancy).

Symptoms and signs
The following 'classical' symptoms and signs are not always present:
- a short period of amenorrhoea (6–8 weeks perhaps)
- unilateral lower abdominal pain
- slight vaginal bleeding arising after the onset of the pain
- shoulder tip pain due to irritation of the diaphragm by blood leaking from the ectopic
- the uterus may be slightly enlarged with cervical excitation and tenderness
- a small tender mass may be palpable to one side of the uterus.
  NB If the history is strongly suggestive of an ectopic pregnancy DO NOT carry out a vaginal examination unless rapid access can be gained to an operating theatre. The tube may rupture, the patient being put at severe risk.

Diagnosis
- Non-rupture of a tubal pregnancy has a positive association with future fertility. Early diagnosis and conservative surgical management are therefore important.
- The diagnosis is not made in 20–25% of cases.
- Even when it is made, the presentation-to-treatment interval is over 48 hours in 40–50%, and over 1 week in 20–25%.
- *When a woman of reproductive age presents with unexplained abdominal pain with or without vaginal bleeding, do not allow home until ectopic pregnancy has been excluded.*

Differential diagnosis
- Threatened or incomplete abortion. In the former there is no pain and in the latter pain follows vaginal bleeding.
- Bleeding corpus luteum—laparoscopy is required to make this differentiation.
- Accident to an ovarian cyst—there is usually no menstrual delay: laparoscopy is indicated.
- Pelvic inflammation—the systemic reaction is more profound and the signs are usually bilateral.

Appropriate intervention must be based on index of suspicion—'think ectopic'.

Investigation
For women in clinically stable conditions with no evidence of intra-abdominal bleeding.

β-hCG estimations using monoclonal antibody tests (which can detect hCG at a level of 1 IU/L).
- If a urine test is positive and an ectopic pregnancy is suspected, carry out a serum assay.
- Most women with ectopic pregnancy have serum β-hCG levels <3000 IU/L. The rate of rise is also important—a doubling time of around 2 days suggests a normally placed pregnancy.

- A negative serum result virtually excludes an ectopic pregnancy, but maintain suspicion if other clinical features are suggestive.
- If the urine or serum test is positive but neither an intra- nor extrauterine pregnancy can be confirmed by ultrasound, repeat test in 48 h.
- The levels of hCG rise more slowly when the pregnancy is extrauterine.

Transvaginal ultrasound. If carried out by properly trained and experienced personnel it may:

- demonstrate an intrauterine pregnancy with no other pelvic pathology (in normal pregnancy a heartbeat can be detected 17 days after the missed period)
- visualise an ectopic, or complex cystic adnexal masses
- show free fluid (blood) in abdomen.

Laparoscopy. The gold standard for diagnosis, indicated if index of suspicion is high. *Very early tubal pregnancies* (3–4% of total) *can still be missed at laparoscopy.*

MANAGEMENT OF ACUTE SITUATION

- If the patient is shocked, laparotomy must be undertaken as quickly as possible.
- The priorities are to stop haemorrhage and prevent further bleeding.
- Conservative surgery is less likely to be possible under these circumstances.

SURGICAL APPROACH IF TUBE UNRUPTURED

Operative laparoscopy is being used increasingly for unruptured ampullary or infundibular pregnancy less than 3 cm in diameter with little or no bleeding into peritoneal cavity (for techniques see Further Reading).

Operative laparoscopy

Potential benefits	*Potential hazards*
• May reduce adhesion formation	• Delayed haemorrhage
• Reduces post-operative stay and convalescence	• Continued trophoblast growth
• Subsequent fertility is at least as good as for laparotomy	

- *It must only be carried out by, or under the direct supervision of, those fully trained in laparoscopic surgery* (see p. 299).
- The preferred conservative procedure is *salpingotomy.*
- Intratubal methotrexate injection after laparoscopic aspiration has been advocated *if there is no haemoperitoneum.*
- The contraindications to conservative laparoscopy are given in the box below.

Absolute contraindications	Relative contraindications
• Patient shocked	• Marked obesity
• Other anaesthetic contraindications to laparoscopy	• Acute and continuing haemorrhage
	• Haematosalpinx >4 cm
• Haematosalpinx >6 cm	• Significant haemoperitoneum
• Serum β-hCG levels >20 000 IU/L	• Dense pelvic adhesions
	• Cornual (interstitial) pregnancy

Salpingectomy can be performed laparoscopically. Results are good in experienced hands. The contraindications are listed in the information box.

Absolute contraindications	Relative contraindications
• Patient shocked	• Marked obesity
• Cornual pregnancy	• Dense pelvic adhesions

Monitor serum β-hCG for at least 2–3 days post-operatively to exclude persistent trophoblast growth.

Laparotomy Conservative surgery should be attempted whenever possible. *Routine salpingectomy is to be deprecated.* Procedures:
- Try to milk the pregnancy from the tube, or
- Carry out a linear salpingostomy along the anti-mesenteric border. The tubal incision can be left open or closed in one or two layers by 6/0 sutures.

CORNUAL (INTERSTITIAL) PREGNANCY

- Although rare, cornual pregnancy can have serious consequences because it is difficult to diagnose early, and when it ruptures it is associated with profuse intraperitoneal bleeding.
- Surgical removal is difficult so injection of methotrexate into the sac laparoscopically or under ultrasound guidance should be considered (see above).

OVARIAN PREGNANCY

To make a diagnosis of primary ovarian pregnancy the following three features must be present:
- the fallopian tube must be intact
- the gestation sac must occupy the anatomical site of the ovary
- ovarian tissue must be demonstrable histologically in the specimen.

ABDOMINAL PREGNANCY

- Both primary and secondary abdominal pregnancies are rare events.
- The fetus may develop fully and survive but the woman usually presents as an acute abdominal emergency in the second trimester.
- It may be possible to make a prospective correct diagnosis if the following features are borne in mind:
  —There is often a history of an episode of abdominal pain and slight vaginal bleeding early in pregnancy, which settled
  —Maternal serum AFP may be elevated
  —The ultrasound scan shows oligohydramnios and no clear uterine outline around the sac. There is also a separate mass related to the gestation sac (this is the uterus).
- When laparotomy is carried out it may not be possible or advisable to remove the placenta because it is likely to be fixed to the abdominal viscera.

CERVICAL PREGNANCY

- This is also rare but may cause profuse vaginal bleeding.
- Hysterectomy may be necessary.
- Injection of methotrexate into the sac is an alternative if the diagnosis is made early enough.

FURTHER READING

Chamberlain G (ed) 1995 Turnbull's obstetrics. Churchill Livingstone, Edinburgh
James D K, Steer P J, Weiner C P, Gonik B (eds) 1994 High risk pregnancy—management options. Saunders, London
Stabile I, Grudzinskas J G 1990 Ectopic pregnancy: a review of incidence, etiology and diagnostic aspects. Obstetrical and Gynecological Survey 45:375–447
Sutton C J S 1989 Laparoscopic surgery. Clinical Obstetrics and Gynaecology 3:429–686

GESTATIONAL TROPHOBLASTIC DISEASE (GTD)

HYDATIDIFORM MOLE (HM)

Molar pregnancies occur in about 1 in 1200 pregnancies. There are two types of hydatidiform mole.

Complete mole (CHM)

The conceptus consists solely of hyperplastic, hydropic chorionic villi; no fetus is present.

- It usually results from fertilisation of an ovum which then loses its nucleus. The haploid sperm duplicates its own chromosomes by meiosis. The result is that:
  —the chromosome complement is usually homozygous 46XX derived solely from the father (androgenetic)
  —only one pair of paternal HLA antigens is expressed.
- About 10% of CHM are heterozygous—usually 46XY but sometimes 46XX. They arise from fertilisation of an anucleate egg by two sperm.
- CHM uniquely combine paternal nuclear DNA with maternal mitochondrial DNA.
- Women with CHM have an increased incidence of balanced translocations and this could explain the loss of the ovum nucleus.

Partial mole (PHM)

There is focal hyperplasia of trophoblast with varying degrees of hydropic villous degeneration; a fetus is present.

- Chromosomal abnormalities (particularly triploidy-69, XXX or XXY) are often found.
- The source of the extra set of chromosomes may be double fertilisation (dispermy) or failure of the first paternal meiotic division.

Risk markers for HM

- *Age*—increased for CHM (but not PHM) at extremes of reproductive life (>30 years and <15 years of age).
- *Ethnic group*—the traditionally reported excess in South-East Asia has decreased and may have been explained by reliance on hospital- rather than population-based data, and greater incidence of pregnancy in young and older women.
- *Previous HM*. The box outlines risk in the next pregnancy.

Number of previous HM	Risk in next pregnancy
1	1:75
2#	1:65

#These women still have a 75% chance of a next successful pregnancy.

- *Previous multiple pregnancy*—twinning and HM may both represent different defects in gametogenesis or fertilisation.

Symptoms
Most are related to excessive production of hCG.
- Amenorrhoea combined with exaggerated pregnancy symptoms, e.g. hyperemesis gravidarum.
- There may be irregular vaginal bleeding that may contain vesicles; many present as incomplete miscarriages.
- Pre-eclampsia may develop unusually early.
- Hyperthyroidism develops in about 5% of women with CHM.
- Rarely massive trophoblastic embolisation may cause respiratory distress requiring prompt treatment (see Further Reading).

Signs
- The uterus may be large for dates.
- Ovaries may be palpably enlarged due to presence of theca-lutein cysts.

Diagnosis
- β-hCG can be markedly raised in serum and urine, but most patients have values within the normal range for pregnancy.
- Ultrasound—the characteristic 'snow-storm' appearance is not pathognomonic. In CHM fetal parts are absent. PHM and missed abortion can be confused.

INVASIVE MOLE (IM)

- There is local invasion of the myometrium and it is therefore much less readily removed by evacuation. The tumour may perforate the uterus. Vaginal metastases may also occur but more distant spread is uncommon.
- This is a histological diagnosis usually made after hysterectomy which has become necessary because vaginal bleeding has continued and hCG levels have remained raised after initial attempts to empty the uterus.
- There is usually a good response to chemotherapy.

PLACENTAL SITE TROPHOBLASTIC TUMOUR (PSTT)

- This is a rare form which appears to arise from placental bed trophoblast rather than the usual villous origin for HM, etc.
- Most cases follow within 3 years of miscarriage or term pregnancy.
- PSTT can be associated with hypertension and the nephrotic syndrome.
- The response to chemotherapy is poor, and hysterectomy is indicated (unless metastasis is advanced).

GESTATIONAL CHORIOCARCINOMA

- This is a highly malignant tumour characterised by disordered growth of syncytio- and cytotrophoblast and invasion of the myometrium causing necrosis and haemorrhage. Metastasis is common.
- It usually arises within 2 years of the causal pregnancy.

Incidence
About 1 in 20 000 to 1 in 40 000 pregnancies in Western countries, increasing to about 1 in 13 000 pregnancies in the Far East.

Risk markers for choriocarcinoma
- Age—as for CHM.
- Obstetric history—only about 1 in 30 hydatidiform moles develop into choriocarcinoma. However, the risk of subsequent choriocarcinoma is 1000 times greater after a mole than after a normal pregnancy. Thus, as many cases follow moles as follow other pregnancies.
- Heterozygous CHM have a greater malignant potential than do homozygous CHM.
- ABO blood group—the risk of choriocarcinoma is increased when the woman and her partner have different ABO groups. Groups B and AB patients have a less good prognosis.
- HLA compatibility between partners may be associated with increased risk of developing choriocarcinoma.

Pathology
- Local extension is frequent but ovarian spread is uncommon.
- The predominant route of spread is vascular. Lymphatic spread is rare.
- Pulmonary metastases occur in about 70% of cases. They may have a 'cannon-ball' or 'snow-storm' appearance or appear intravascular on chest X-ray. Haemoptysis is a common symptom.

STAGING OF GTD

Stage	Disease development
0	Molar pregnancy
I	Persistently elevated β-hCG titres (i.e. 6 months or more after evacuation) and tumour confined to body of uterus
II	Pelvic and/or vaginal metastasis
III	Pulmonary metastasis
IV	All other distant metastases

A prognostic scoring system can be used in Stages I–IV to determine the appropriate treatment for each patient. (For details see Further Reading.) It is based on:
- the extent of the tumour burden, e.g. β-hCG level, and number, site and size of metastases
- patient characteristics, e.g. risk increases with age and parity
- the nature of and the interval since the antecedent pregnancy: the risk is highest for a term pregnancy and lowest for a hydatidiform mole. The longer the interval, the higher the risk
- the patient's ability to respond immunologically, e.g. a well-developed lymphocytic infiltrate around the tumour is a favourable feature
- ABO blood groups of both partners
- poor response to previous chemotherapy.

MANAGEMENT OF GTD

Stage 0
- Once a firm diagnosis is made the mole needs to be removed, preferably by suction evacuation and curettage.
- This may need to be repeated if:
  —irregular bleeding persists, or
  —β-hCG levels are still elevated 6 weeks after initial evacuation. Hysterectomy can be carried out in older women whose family is complete.
- In the UK, patients should be registered with one of the three reference laboratories—London, Sheffield and Dundee.
- Follow-up—serum β-hCG estimations should be carried out weekly until levels are normal (<5 IU/L). If that happens within 6 weeks, tests are continued monthly for 6 months.
  —If serum β-hCG levels take longer than 8 weeks to become normal, follow up monthly for 1 year and then 3-monthly during the second year
  —The patient may begin to try to become pregnant 6 months after β-hCG values have become and remain normal
  —A barrier method of contraception should be used until β-hCG levels are normal: then oral contraception can be used
  —There may be a higher incidence of subsequent choriocarcinoma if the 'pill' is started before hCG levels fall
  —β-hCG levels should be checked 3 weeks after the end of any pregnancy subsequent to a molar pregnancy.

Stages I–IV
- The disease progresses in <10% of affected women. Among the indications that chemotherapy may be necessary are:
  —β-hCG levels remain markedly elevated 6 weeks after evacuation
  —β-hCG levels remain the same for 3 successive months or begin to rise again

—persistent or recurrent uterine bleeding with raised β-hCG
  levels.
* Management of Stages I–IV should be confined to specialised
  centres (see Further Reading).

Results of therapy
Remission can be expected in all women adequately treated in
Stages I–III and in up to 70% of women with Stage IV disease.

Subsequent pregnancies
* A normal outcome can be expected.
* The incidence of congenital malformation does not seem to be
  increased in women who have received chemotherapy.

FURTHER READING

Chamberlain G (ed) 1995 Turnbull's obstetrics. Churchill Livingstone, Edinburgh
James D K, Steer P J, Weiner C P, Gonik B (eds) 1994 High risk pregnancy—
  management options. Saunders, London

4. Congenital abnormalities

Malformation
• A primary error in normal development of an organ or tissue.

Disruption
• A secondary malformation resulting from damage to a previously normal organ or tissue.
• About 15% of newborns have a single minor malformation.
• Major congenital malformations constitute 10% of miscarriages, 3% of all deliveries, under 2% of livebirths, and about 30% of all stillbirths, neonatal deaths and infant deaths.
• The incidence is more than doubled in multiple pregnancy (especially in monozygotic twins).
• Perinatal mortality due to malformations is around 2.5/1000 births: 30% of all children born alive with major malformations die within 5 years.
• The information box gives the approximate birth incidence of major malformations.

Major malformations: approximate birth incidence	
CNS 10/1000 births	Limbs 2/1000 births
CVS 8/1000 births	Others 6/1000 births
Renal tract 4/1000 births	**Total** 30/1000 births

Deformation
• An alteration in shape or position due to inappropriate mechanical forces.
• The most significant are congenital dislocation of the hip (CDH) and talipes equinovarus.
• Deformations can have intrinsic or extrinsic causes and can be associated with:
  —neuromuscular or connective tissue disorders
  —CNS malformation (intrinsic)
  —oligohydramnios, malpresentations, uterine anomalies and multiple pregnancy (extrinsic).
• About 2% of newborns are affected; one third of these have multiple deformations.

AETIOLOGY

The most important causes of congenital defects and their approximate incidence are given in the information box.

Cause	Incidence
Idiopathic	60%
'Multifactorial'	20%
Single-gene disorders	7–8%
Chromosomal	6%
Infections	2%
Maternal illness (e.g. epilepsy, diabetes)	3%
Drugs, radiation, alcohol	1–2%

GENETICS

Major increases in knowledge have occurred in this field over the last decade, and will continue. Scientists, doctors and society in general have hardly begun to consider the ethical and practical implications of this information explosion.

Cytogenetics
- The normal human karyotype has 46 chromosomes: 22 pairs of autosomes, and 2 sex chromosomes—XX in the normal female and XY in the normal male.
- Each chromosome has:
  —a *centromere*—the narrow waist which may be near the middle (metacentric), close to one end (acrocentric), or in an intermediate position (submetacentric)
  —a long arm (q) and a short arm (p)
  —a *telomere* at the tip of each arm.

Mitosis
A process by which all somatic cells divide.
- It involves splitting of each of the 46 chromosomes to provide a full identical (diploid) complement for both daughter cells.
- It is divided into five stages:
  —*Interphase*—the period between successive cell divisions
  —*Prophase*—the chromatids split longitudinally into pairs of chromatids connected at the centromere
  —*Metaphase*—movement of the chromatids occurs towards the equator of the cell
  —*Anaphase*—the centromeres divide, and the paired chromatids separate
  —*Telophase*—the cytoplasm divides, the chromosomes unwind, and two genetically identical daughter cells are formed.

Meiosis

A process by which all germ cells (gametes) divide and during which the chromosome of the daughter cells is halved (haploid). Two sequential cell divisions are involved:

- interchange or cross-over of chromosomal material can take place during prophase of the first division; daughter cells inherit chromatid pairs still attached at the centromere
- completion of separation.

Summary

- The somatic cell produces, by mitosis, two diploid cells, each containing 46 chromosomes.
- The germ cell produces, by meiosis, four haploid gametes, each with 23 chromosomes.
- Gametogenesis is discussed on page 202.

CHROMOSOMAL DISORDERS

- 95% of gametes with chromosome abnormalities are not viable.
- They affect at least 7% of all conceptions and 6/1000 of all livebirths.
- They are present in 60% of first-trimester miscarriages, 5% of second-trimester miscarriages, and 4–5% of stillbirths.
- Abnormalities can be numerical or structural.

NUMERICAL ABERRATIONS

Aneuploidy

An abnormality in number of chromosomes, usually by mutation.

- It can arise during meiosis or mitosis.
- It is usually due to the failure of paired chromosomes to separate at anaphase (non-disjunction), or their delayed movement at the same stage (anaphase lag).
- Two cells are produced, one with an extra copy of a chromosome (trisomy), the other with that chromosome missing (monosomy).

Polyploidy

The number of chromosomes is an exact multiple of the haploid, but greater than the diploid number, e.g. triploidy (69XXY is the most common), or tetraploidy (4n).

STRUCTURAL ABERRATIONS

Due to chromosome breakage and inappropriate rejoining of the broken ends.

- *Translocation* of fragments between chromosomes—there are three types:
  —reciprocal, in which the chromosomal material distal to breaks in two chromosomes is exchanged

—Robertsonian, in which breaks in two acrocentric chromosomes (most commonly numbers 13 and 14) occur near the centromere with cross-fusion of the products
—insertional, in which three breaks occur in one or two chromosomes often inherited.
- A *balanced translocation* exists when the genome contains the correct amount of genetic matter, and they usually have no outward manifestation. Parental karyotyping is essential. If one parent has a balanced translocation the theoretical outlook for any offspring is: 1:4 have the same balanced translocation; 1:4 have normal chromosomes; 1:2 have an unbalanced translocation.
- *Unbalanced translocations*
  —The origin rather than the new site is of greater importance
  —If the chromosomal anomaly is large enough to be seen under the microscope it is likely to involve enough chromatin to cause major problems
  —Malformations are usual and mental retardation invariable
  —Parental karyotyping will identify a balanced rearrangement.
- *Deletion*—loss of any part of a chromosome.
  —Substantial losses are nearly always lethal
  —A *ring chromosome* can result if both arms of a chromosome break, the terminal ends are lost, and the two proximal sticky ends unite.
- *Duplication*—two copies of a chromosome segment are present.
  —It is more common than deletion but generally less harmful.
- *Inversion*—two breaks occur in one chromosome with inversion of 180° of the segment between breaks.
  —It does not usually produce a clinical abnormality but can give rise to unbalanced gametes.
- *Isochromosome*—deletion of one and duplication of the other chromosome.
  —The commonest in livebirths is that of the long arm of X which is a cause of Turner's syndrome (p. 246).

OTHER ABERRATIONS

- *Mosaic*—an individual with two or more cell lines derived from a single zygote
- *Chimaera*—two cell lines are derived from two separate zygotes. It can arise by:
  —early fusion of dizygotic twin zygotes
  —double fertilisation of the egg and a polar body
  —exchange of haemopoietic cells in utero between dizygotic twins.

AUTOSOMAL ABNORMALITIES

DOWN'S SYNDROME

- The overall incidence is about 1/650 livebirths.
- Between 65 and 80% of affected fetuses miscarry or are stillborn.
- Genetic abnormalities are listed in the box.

Genetic abnormalities in Down's syndrome	
• Trisomy 21 (due to non-disjunction)	95%
• Translocation 14:21	2%
• Other translocations	2%
• Mosaicism	1%

- The maternal risk of trisomy 21 is age-related, being 1/1530 at 20 years rising to 1/37 at 44 years.
- The risk of recurrence of Down's syndrome due to trisomy 21 is about 1/100.
- For mothers aged 35 years or over, the risk of Down's syndrome or another chromosomal abnormality recurring is approximately four times the age-related risk.
- The risk of translocation 14:21 recurring is about 1/10 if the mother has a balanced translocation; 1/50 if the father has it.

Effects of Down's syndrome

- Newborns are often 'small for dates' and hypotonic.
- Facies are characteristically 'mongoloid'.
- Affected children are often happy and affectionate.
- Mean IQ is 40–50 (moderate disability) with a range of 20 (severe) to 70 (mild).
- Associated complications include congenital heart disease (40%); duodenal atresia (<10%); and leukaemia (1%).
- Many develop Alzheimer's disease in later life.

Biochemical screening for Down's syndrome

- Even if all pregnant women aged 35 years or over elected to have an amniocentesis, this would result in a detection rate for Down's syndrome of 35% for an amniocentesis rate of 7.5%.
- Detection rates are increased by measuring AFP, unconjugated oestriol (E_3), and hCG at 15–18 weeks and calculating a maternal age-specific related risk of Down's syndrome. AFP and E_3 tend to be reduced and hCG increased in affected pregnancies.
- At a risk cut-off level of 1 in 200, biochemical screening raises the detection level to 60% with an amniocentesis rate of 5% and a 4.5% false-positive rate.
- *The anxiety induced by a false-positive diagnosis must not be underestimated.*

- Mothers must be enabled to make a properly informed choice to 'opt in' to the programme.
- The programme must be adequately resourced to include counselling for those found to be at 'high risk'.
- In some cases ultrasound examination may raise the index of suspicion by observing subtle markers such as nuchal oedema (see p. 50).

TRISOMY 13 (PATAU'S) AND 18 (EDWARDS') SYNDROME

- Also maternal age-related: due to non-disjunction
- Both universally lethal, usually in the neonatal period
- Cleft lip and palate, renal and other malformations (e.g. holoprosencephaly in t13) and IUGR are usual
- Recurrence risk is probably low.

TRIPLOIDY

- Survival to livebirth is rare with subsequent neonatal death associated with severe IUGR and multiple malformations.
- Elongation of second digit and syndactyly of third/fourth digit is characteristic.

Table 4.1   Sex chromosome disorders

Defect	Incidence compared with livebirths	Average IQ	Association with maternal age
XO	1:3000 (1:100 conceptions)	100	Incidence falls as age rises
XXX	1:1000	Possible slight reduction	Increased × 2–3 when maternal age >40
XXY	1:700	100	Increased × 2–3 when maternal age >40
XYY	1:700	100	None

- These conditions have a much better outlook than was originally thought (for further discussion see pp. 246–249).
- Antenatal detection does not necessarily warrant termination of pregnancy.
- About 5% of XO females will have periods and a few may be fertile.

COMMON SINGLE-GENE DISORDERS
AUTOSOMAL DOMINANT CONDITIONS

- These are often mild (e.g. polydactyly), have various degrees of manifestation or, if severe, arise during adulthood (e.g. polycystic kidneys) or at the end of the reproductive period (e.g. Huntington's chorea).
- The combined incidence of all dominants is 7/1000 livebirths.
- 50% of the offspring of an affected individual will be affected.
- Counselling is complicated by variable expression and incomplete penetrance which cause the various degrees of manifestation.
- The commonest dominant condition is *familial hypercholesterolaemia* (up to 1/250 of the population).

Myotonic dystrophy
Caused by a gene defect on chromosome 19q.
- It is important because of its incidence (approx. 1/5000); variability of expression with increased severity in each subsequent generation; increased subfertility and anaesthetic risks in those affected.
- If a mother has symptomatic myotonic dystrophy the condition may present in utero with reduced fetal movement, polyhydramnios and pre-term delivery of a baby who has contractures, hypotonia and respiratory and feeding difficulties.
- A direct and specific DNA test is available for pre-pregnancy and prenatal testing if:
  —there is a family history of myotonic dystrophy
  —either parent is affected
  —a previous child had congenital myotonic dystrophy.

Huntington's chorea
Caused by a gene defect on chromosome 4p.
- Although rare, its effects are devastating and there is no treatment.
- The symptoms of involuntary movement, depression and dementia usually commence between 30 and 60 years of age.
- DNA testing is available for diagnosis in symptomatic cases.
- Its use for prenatal testing is highly controversial because of the major implications of a positive test for a presymptomatic parent.

Prenatal testing
Can be offered for many other dominant conditions by DNA analysis from CVS.
- In most cases at present this relies on linked polymorphic DNA markers which require prior family studies—e.g. adult polycystic kidneys, familial retinoblastoma or Marfan's syndrome.

- Diagnosis by direct mutation detection is increasingly possible—
  e.g. peroneal muscular atrophy, retinitis pigmentosa (some
  families) or familial polyposis coli.

AUTOSOMAL RECESSIVE CONDITIONS

- The gene must be inherited from both parents.
- The effects are usually severe.
- 50% of offspring of affected individuals will be carriers.
- Consanguineous couples have an increased risk depending on
  closeness of relationship and family history (FH).
  —If there is no significant FH the risk in offspring of first cousins
    is 5% (cf. 2% background risk)
  —Offer prenatal diagnosis if both partners are carriers or carrier
    status cannot be determined.

Cystic fibrosis (CF)
The commonest recessive condition in the UK.
- 1/22 persons are carriers (heterozygotes).
- 1/500 couples are at a 1/4 risk of having an affected child.
- The CF gene is located on chromosome 7 (region 7q32).
- One mutation (ΔF508) causes 70% of all faulty CF genes in the
  UK.
- Adults with CF are usually subfertile (males may be sterile).

Presentation
- CF typically presents in childhood with failure to thrive, recurrent
  chest infection and malabsorption.
- The fetus or neonate may have meconium ileus or peritoneal
  calcification.
- The risk of pre-term delivery and maternal and perinatal
  mortality may be increased.
- Affected mothers are at risk from cardiorespiratory failure—
  regular antenatal assessment is necessary. Women with severe
  respiratory impairment should be strongly advised to avoid
  pregnancy.

Table 4.2 Testing for cystic fibrosis

Index pregnancy	One affected parent	Couple with previous CF child	Family history or one parent with CF child by different partner	Fetus with meconium ileus or peritoneal calcification
Risk of CF	1/44	1/4	Risk depends on closeness of relationship	Diagnostic tests needed
Pre-pregnancy	Screen *both* parents for DNA mutations	Screen DNA from affected child and both parents	Screen DNA from both parents	
Antenatal	Offer CVS* at 11 weeks only if partner has a CF mutation (because risk of CF in fetus now 1/2)	Offer CVS* at 11 weeks if both parents carry a mutation, otherwise discuss with geneticist	Offer CVS* if both parents carry a mutation (risk now 1/4)	Obtain DNA from CVS*: if both parents carry a mutation, diagnosis confirmed: check alkaline phosphatase in 16–19 wk amniocentesis if only 1 or 0 mutations found

* chorionic villus sampling

Other recessive disorders
- Most serious disorders are very rare (<1/40 000) and carrier frequency is low (<1/100).
- For parents with a previously affected child the recurrence risk is 1/4.
- Prenatal diagnosis is by CVS—biochemical analysis for metabolic disorders; DNA analysis is available for an increasing number of others (consult geneticist).
- Prior DNA studies on parents and affected child are required to discover how informative testing will be.
- In different racial groups some recessive conditions are more frequent and prenatal testing is as for CF in Caucasians, e.g.:
  —thalassaemias in Asian, African and Mediterranean populations
  —sickle cell disease in Afro-Caribbean population
  —Tay–Sachs in Ashkenazi Jews.

Thalassaemias
Autosomal recessively inherited defects in the rate of synthesis of one or more globin chains.
- α-thalassaemia is due to the deletion of structural DNA genes affecting the α-Hb chains.
- HbF contains α chains, therefore the fetus can be affected to an extent varying from anaemia to hydrops.
- β-thalassaemia is due to a messenger RNA abnormality causing defective production of β-Hb chains:
  —β+ disease—reduced production of β chains
  —β0 disease—no β chains.
- In β0 and β+ disease homozygotes are affected severely (thalassaemia major) from which up to 100 000 children die world-wide each year.
- In high-risk population, screen before pregnancy by full blood count, film and Hb electrophoresis.
- If both parents are carriers for same type, check blood for DNA mutations.
- If both parents carry the mutation, offer CVS for DNA testing or check globin chain synthesis by fetal blood sampling (see p. 51).
- If previous child affected, offer CVS as above.

Sickle cell disease
- This is due to structural alterations in one of the globin chains.
  —There are more than 80 α chains and 180 β chain variants; the most important clinically are HbS and HbC
  —HbS/S is commonest and most troublesome in tropical Africa (heterozygote frequency 20–40%). It is also present among North American Blacks (heterozygote frequency 9%), in the Middle East, India and the Mediterranean littoral
  —HbS/C affects West Indian Black populations particularly severely.

- The high world-wide frequency of the sickle cell and thalassaemia genes probably occurs because heterozygotes are protected against falciparum malaria.
- Screen for carrier status by 'sickle test' in Afro-Caribbean population.
- Direct DNA testing is available for fetus—the sickle cell mutation alters a 'restriction enzyme chopping site' in the β-globin gene.

Phenylketonuria (PKU)
- The gene defect is on chromosome 12q. Carrier detection and prenatal diagnosis in affected families is now possible using direct DNA testing.
- Routine neonatal screening is still mandatory.
- A mother with PKU has about an 8% chance of having an affected child.
- She must receive a phenylalanine-free diet from before conception; otherwise the risk of spontaneous abortion, infant death or severe mental retardation is high, even if the child has not inherited the disorder.

X-LINKED RECESSIVE DISORDERS

- An initial guide to carrier status is based on family studies plus clinical, biochemical or haematological tests.
- More definitive information is obtained from DNA studies. In most cases this is by analysis of indirect linked markers but an increasing number of individual gene mutations are being discovered which can be analysed directly.
- Prenatal diagnosis should be considered only after full evaluation of carrier status by a clinical geneticist and by prior consideration of what can/should be done with the information.

Duchenne/Becker muscular dystrophies (DMD/BMD)
- Boys with DMD may present with delayed onset of walking (i.e. after 18 months), with progressive muscular weakness and death from cardio-respiratory failure by 25 years. BMD is milder, progressing to wheelchair use by 45 years.
- 1/3000 males are born with a mutation in the dystrophin gene at *Xp21* resulting in either DMD or BMD.
- 1/2000 women are carriers—a few may have mild symptoms (or very rarely the full disease due to X-autosome translocation or as a monozygous twin).
- Fresh mutation accounts for one third of boys with DMD (i.e. two thirds of mothers are carriers): a higher proportion of BMD mothers are carriers.

Pre-pregnancy screening for DMD/BMD
- Indicated if previously affected son or family history of DMD or BMD

- Direct DNA testing is possible in the 70% of families with a readily detectable dystrophin gene mutation. Indirect DNA testing is used for the remaining 30%
- If the male partner is affected check his DNA for deletion in dystrophin gene. Prenatal testing is not indicated—no son will be affected but all daughters will be carriers.

Prenatal diagnosis of DMD/BMD
- Offer CVS if dystrophin gene deletion found in above. Otherwise discuss with geneticist
- Ethical debate continues about investigation and reporting of carrier state in female fetus.

Fragile X-associated mental retardation The second commonest genetic cause of mental retardation (after Down's syndrome).
- Due to mutation in *FraX* gene at tip of X chromosome
- Incidence is 1/2500 males
- About one third of female carriers have mental retardation (usually milder than in affected males)
- Prenatal DNA testing now possible
- Antenatal screening cannot yet be justified and needs further study
- Referral to clinical geneticist essential in presence of FH of condition.

Other X-linked recessive disorders e.g. *Haemophilia A* (factor VIII deficiency affecting 1/5000 males) or *Haemophilia B* (factor IX deficiency affecting 1/30 000 males) should be approached as above.

MULTIFACTORIAL DISORDERS

The most significant conditions within this group are neural tube defects, many congenital heart lesions, facial clefts, diaphragmatic herniae, and gut atresias.

NEURAL TUBE DEFECTS (NTD)

- Anencephaly and spina bifida comprise 95% of NTDs and encephalocele the remaining 5%.
- The incidence is inversely related to socioeconomic status and shows marked geographical variation (ranging from 3/1000 births in SE England to 8–10/1000 in Ireland).
- Incidence has dropped steadily over the past 20 years—this is not entirely accounted for by antenatal screening programmes.
- In the UK the recurrence risk after one affected child is 1 in 25, rising to 1 in 10 after two or more. An affected parent has a 1 in 25 risk of producing a child with a NTD.

Screening for NTD

- This has relied on a cut-off level for maternal serum α-fetoprotein (AFP) of around 2.5 multiples of the normal median (MoM) at 16–18 weeks' gestation which detects 90% of anencephaly, 80% of open spina bifida, but will include 3% of unaffected singleton pregnancies.
- Results at least as good as these are now being obtained using high-resolution ultrasound imaging carried out by properly trained personnel (see p. 8).

Prevention of NTD

The risk of recurrence may be reduced if multivitamin tablets, which include folic acid (400 μg daily), are taken from at least 1 month before conception to about 8 weeks of pregnancy.

AFP and other fetal problems

- High serum AFP levels may be associated with conditions such as exomphalos, congenital nephrosis, posterior urethral valves, Turner's syndrome and trisomy 13.
- High serum AFP alone predicts an increased risk of a variety of obstetric problems, including IUGR and perinatal death, particularly if oligohydramnios is present.

CONGENITAL HEART LESIONS

- The overall incidence has inexplicably increased over the past 15 years and is now about 8/1000 births.
- The incidence and recurrence risks for various types of congenital heart defects are given in Table 4.3.
- Prenatal diagnosis of some of the most serious of the defects is possible using high-resolution ultrasound imaging and fetal echocardiography at 20 weeks' gestation (see p. 50).

Table 4.3 Congenital heart lesions: incidence and recurrence risks

Defect	Birth incidence	Recurrence risk for sibs	Recurrence risk for offspring
Ventricular septal defect	1/400	1 in 25	1 in 25
Atrial septal defect	1/1000	1 in 33	1 in 33
Tetralogy of Fallot	1/1000	1 in 33	1 in 25
Coarctation of aorta	1/1600	1 in 50	1 in 50
Aortic stenosis	1/2000	1 in 50	1 in 33
Transposition of the great vessels	1/16 000	1 in 50	unknown

FACIAL CLEFTS

- Cleft lip and/or palate occurs in 1/1000 births.
- Most are multifactorial but it is associated with over 150 rare single-gene traits or chromosomal abnormalities (e.g. trisomy 13).
- Surgical repair with good results is usual.
- Recurrence risks for the multifactorial lesions are:
  —child with unilateral cleft lip in normal parents: 1 in 50
  —child with bilateral cleft lips and palate in normal parents: 1 in 20.
- Isolated cleft palate is distinct. It affects 1 in 2500 births, with a recurrence risk of 1 in 50 for sibs and offspring.

ANTERIOR ABDOMINAL WALL DEFECTS

These occur in about 1/6000 pregnancies, and the two main forms are:
- *exomphalos*—the umbilical cord is involved and is attached to the apex of the sac which may contain liver and/or intestines. Associated chromosomal anomalies occur in 30% and cardiac lesions in 10%
- *gastroschisis*—the umbilical cord is not involved and there is no sac. Associated gut atresias and cardiac lesions (but not chromosome abnormalities) occur in up to 20%
  —Prenatal diagnosis by ultrasound is possible
  —Maternal serum AFP may be elevated

Chromosomal anomalies should be excluded if exomphalos is suspected.
Vaginal delivery should be aimed for except for obstetric indications.
Isolated defects are often correctable surgically.
Body stalk anomalies form a third, less common defect. They are associated with major lower body deformities.

GASTROINTESTINAL ANOMALIES

Among those with multifactorial inheritance patterns are:
- *Hirschsprung's disease*—affects 1/8000 newborns with a 3-to-1 male excess.

Table 4.4 Hirschsprung's disease: recurrence risk

	Sibs	Offspring
Affected male	1 in 25	<1 in 100
Affected female	1 in 8	<1 in 100

- *Pyloric stenosis*—incidence 1/200 in males and 1/1000 in females.
  —The greatest risk of recurrence is in male relatives of an affected female (1/6)
  —The lowest risk is for female relatives of an affected male (1/50)
  —The risks for the other two possible combinations are intermediate.
- *Oesophageal atresia/tracheo-oesophageal fistulae*—affect 1/3000 newborns.
  —May be associated with cardiac defects
  —Can be suspected prenatally by persistent absence of stomach bubble on ultrasound.
- *Gut atresias*—affect 1/330 newborns and may occur at any level of the intestine.
  —Can be diagnosed prenatally by ultrasound.
- *Diaphragmatic herniae*—occur in 1/2000 to 1/5000 births: 95% of affected fetuses are stillborn.
  —The incidence of associated anomalies may be as high as 60% overall.

OTHER MALFORMATIONS

Obstructive uropathies—dilatation of whole or part of urinary tract is most commonly due to *urethral valves.*
- This affects males 20 times more often than females.
- The prognosis depends on the time of onset and severity of the obstruction.
- The dilated urinary tract can be observed ultrasonically in the fetus.
- The role of fetal therapy is discussed on page 52.

GENETIC COUNSELLING AND PRENATAL DIAGNOSIS

Ethical issues Knowledge about and techniques for studying fetal development in general and genetics in particular are advancing rapidly.
- This increases our responsibility to consider the ethical issues raised. 'What *can* we do?' must be balanced by 'What *ought* we to do?'

- Among the ethical dilemmas we face are:
  - —general population screening for defective genes, e.g. the cystic fibrosis gene
  - —testing of pre-implantation embryos after assisted conception
  - —more aggressive prenatal screening for conditions causing varying degrees of disability, e.g. Down's syndrome
  - —false-positive rates inherent in all screening programmes.

Genetic counselling is the imparting of knowledge and advice about inherited conditions. This involves:

- complete history from or about the affected individual (proband)
- construction of pedigree
- physical examination of proband with particular reference to dysmorphic features
- accurate diagnosis—the indications for chromosome analysis are given in the box
- non-directive counselling
- follow-up.

Indications for chromosome analysis

- Family history of chromosomal aberration
- Multiple congenital anomalies
- Unexplained short stature in female
- Unexplained stillbirth
- Some forms of cancer associated with chromosomal rearrangements

- Dysmorphic features
- Ambiguous genitalia
- Unexplained mental retardation
- Recurrent miscarriage
- Neuroblastoma, leukaemia, retinoblastoma, Wilm's tumour

Prenatal diagnosis

- Can be justified if the condition:
  - —is severe in its effects
  - —has a high genetic risk
  - —is untreatable.
- The test must be reliable, and must be preceded by counselling.
- Tests for those anomalies which can be diagnosed antenatally can be applied:
  - —as a *screening test* in a whole population to define a subgroup at particular risk with whom diagnostic procedures can be discussed
  - —as *diagnostic tests* in a group of women at high risk of a particular problem, e.g. a previous personal or family history of chromosomal disorders or inborn errors of metabolism: women with 'positive' screening tests

- The basis of diagnosis is either:
  —the search for characteristic intracellular defects in fetal tissue obtained by invasive procedures (see below), or
  —the visualisation of morphological defects by ultrasound.

DIAGNOSTIC TECHNIQUES

Ultrasonography

- This has become the main diagnostic technique for prenatal diagnosis of congenital anomalies by allowing:
  —direct visualisation of the defect, e.g. anencephaly
  —detection of markers of chromosomal defects
  —accurate direction of instruments during invasive procedures.
- The best time for routine examination is 18–20 weeks.
- Detailed ultrasound requires great interpretative skill from the operator if unacceptable levels of false-positive and false-negative diagnosis are to be avoided.
- Some of the more sophisticated techniques should be carried out in regional centres with the appropriate expertise.
- Table 4.5 highlights some specific points. For more detailed discussion see Further Reading.

Table 4.5 Ultrasonography in prenatal diagnosis

Condition	Ultrasonic examination	Comment
Spina bifida	Bi-parietal diameter (BPD) and head circumference reduced; ventriculomegaly; scalloping of frontal bones ('lemon sign'); anterior curve of cerebellar hemispheres ('banana sign') or absent cerebellum (all at 16–18 weeks)	Reliable when examined by experienced personnel. The presence of some of these signs indicates need for more detailed examination
Congenital heart defects	'Four chamber' view of heart at transverse section of thorax	Optimum time for examination: 18–24 weeks
	Echocardiography for individual women at high risk	For specialised centres only
Down's syndrome	Ratio of bi-parietal to occipito-frontal diameter to detect brachycephaly	Of no value in population screening
	Nuchal skin thickness	May occur in normal fetuses; varies with attitude of fetal head; can be produced artificially by angle of transducer
	Short femur (using increased BPD: femur length ratio as index)	May be useful as ancillary screening method at 16 weeks

Chorionic villus (CV) biopsy

- CV biopsy obtains fetal tissue from the chorion under ultrasound guidance.
- One technique uses a transcervical approach between 8 and 12 weeks. The second, and now more popular, transabdominal route can be used from 8 weeks to term.
- The additional procedure-related risk of miscarriage is about 2%.
- Its potential advantages are:
  —it can be carried out in the first trimester
  —the tissue is ideal for DNA analysis and gene probing (see below)
  —initial chromosome analysis can be ready in about 48 hours (full cultures still take 2–3 weeks).
- However, the genetic composition of the chorion (trophoblast) is not necessarily the same as that of the fetus. For example, mosaicism and some rare trisomies confined to the trophoblast occur in about 1% of cases.
- *Chromosomal aberrations found after CV biopsy must therefore be assessed carefully.*

Amniocentesis

This is best carried out at 15–18 weeks' gestation. The failure rate is <1%. The average time for culture is 10–12 days.

Indications
- Maternal request based on age-related risk or screening test
- Previous infant affected by a condition diagnosable antenatally
- Family or personal history of diagnosable condition.

Risks
- Miscarriage—the excess procedure-related risk is between 0.5 and 1%. It is related to experience and use of ultrasound guidance.

Precautions
- Always use ultrasound to continuously observe the needle during the procedure.
- Give anti-D immunoglobulin 50 µg in all antibody-negative, Rh-D-negative women and to those whose Rh group is unknown. More can be given to cover any serious feto-maternal transfusion (see p. 93).

Fetal blood sampling (cordocentesis)

- The sample is taken under ultrasonic guidance from the area of the insertion of the cord into the placenta.
- *It must be carried out only in specialist centres.*
- Among the indications are red-cell immunisation (see p. 93); non-immune hydrops (see p. 123); exclusion of fetal infection (see p. 106); and rapid karyotyping in some cases of IUGR (see p. 60).

- Anti-D immunoglobulin (100 µg, or more if Kleihauer indicates it) should be given to Rh-D-negative women carrying Rh-D-positive fetuses.
- The risk of fetal loss is about 1%.

Embryo biopsy

- IVF and embryo culture allow sampling of one or two cells at 8 to 16-cell stage.
- DNA analysis of a single cell and/or karyotyping of cultured cell could be used for diagnosis of genetic defect in women at high risk of a serious disorder.
- Only normal embryos would be reimplanted.
- This is potentially more acceptable for some couples than later prenatal diagnostic methods.
- It could ultimately allow 'gene therapy' in some cases.
- However, even if the embryos are 'normal' the rate of successful pregnancies will be reduced.

FETAL THERAPY

- This can be achieved indirectly via the mother (e.g digoxin or flecainide for fetal cardiac arrhythmias) or directly to the fetus, as listed in the information box.

Therapy direct to the fetus

Medical
Intravascular infusions or injections by cordocentesis for

- Transfusion to correct anaemia, e.g. for iso-immunisation
- Platelet infusion injection for allo-immune thrombocytopenia (see p. 000)
- Drug injection, e.g. to treat fetal hypothyroidism or cardiac failure

Surgical
Ultrasound-guided techniques can be used to

- Drain pleural effusions or ascites
- Insert pleuro-amniotic shunts for non-immune hydrops or chylothorax
- Insert vesico-amniotic shunts to relieve obstructive uropathies. No consensus exists about criteria for this. In selected cases decompression may restore amniotic fluid volume and prevent pulmonary hypoplasia. It is unlikely to prevent or reverse renal damage

---

- *Fetal karyotyping should be considered before therapeutic interventions are carried out.*

POST-MORTEM EXAMINATION OF FETUSES

- An experienced perinatal pathologist should be asked to examine all mid-trimester spontaneous abortions and those induced because of suspected congenital malformations.
- This will allow accurate counselling of the families, and audit of the screening and diagnostic tests (see also p. 9).

FURTHER READING

Chamberlain G (ed) 1995 Turnbull's obstetrics. Churchill Livingstone, Edinburgh

Creasy R K, Resnik R (eds) 1994 Maternal–fetal medicine—principles and practice, 3rd edn. Saunders, Philadelphia

James D K, Steer P J, Weiner C P, Gonik B (eds) 1994 High risk pregnancy—management options. Saunders, London

Rosevear S K, Stirrat G M 1996 Handbook of obstetric management. Blackwell Scientific, Oxford

RCOG Working Party on Biochemical Markers and the Detection of Down's Syndrome 1993: Report. RCOG, London

RCOG/RCGP 1995 Guidance on ultrasound procedures in early pregnancy. RCOG/RCGP, London

5. Assessment of fetal growth and well-being

NORMAL FETAL GROWTH

- Fetal growth and fetal size are often confused in clinical practice (see below).
- The average weights of normal fetuses as pregnancy progresses are given in the box.

Average weights of normal fetuses	
Gestational age (weeks)	Approx. weight (grams)
10	5
20	300
30	1500
40	3400

- About 95% of birthweights fall within a normal distribution curve but the remaining 5% show a prolonged tail of low birthweight which is discussed below.

FACTORS AFFECTING FETAL GROWTH AND SIZE

Physiological

Genetic control
- This predominates in the first half of pregnancy, but environmental factors and other constraints give rise to greater variability in the second half of pregnancy.
- About 15% of total birthweight variation is attributable to the fetal genotype.

Fetal sex
- On average males weigh 150–200 g more than females at term.
- There is no difference up to 33 weeks' gestation.

Race. The approximate mean birthweight for six ethnic groups are given in the box.

Ethnic group	Approx. mean birthweight
Europeans	3200 g
East and South-west Asians	3100 g
Indonesians and Africans	3000 g
Indians	2900 g

These differences do not solely depend on race; nutritional and socioeconomic factors are likely to be involved.

Parental height and weight
- The paternal contribution is solely genetic.
- Maternal height and weight have independent effects on birthweight.
- Tall, heavy mothers will have babies up to 500 g heavier than short, light mothers.

Maternal age. Teenage mothers and those over 35 years of age tend to have smaller babies (as well as an increased incidence of congenital anomaly). Socioeconomic factors also play a role.

Birth order. Birthweight rises from first to second pregnancies by about 130 g, with a smaller rise in the third pregnancy. This may be associated with increased maternal weight.

Multiple pregnancy. Twin growth is similar to singletons up to 32 weeks but decreases thereafter. Dizygotic twins tend to be heavier than monozygotic. No weight-for-gestation standards exist for multiple pregnancy.

Socioeconomic
- The average birthweight of babies born into social classes I and II (professional and managerial) is 150 g greater than for babies born into social classes IV and V. This may be related to maternal size, age and smoking habits rather than to nutritional status.
- In general, the growing fetus is protected against the effects of maternal deprivation unless they are very severe.

Pathological markers for reduced fetal growth
- *Previous obstetric history.* Women whose first pregnancy ended in stillbirth (but not miscarriage), or in birth of a growth-retarded baby, tend to have relatively small babies in subsequent pregnancies.

- *Smoking and altitude.* Smoking in pregnancy reduces the mean birthweight by 100–200 g from 34 weeks' gestation onwards. Birthweight falls by about 100 g for every 1000 metres of altitude.
- Excessive alcohol ingestion (see p. 63).
- Pre-eclampsia and related disorders.
- Congenital malformation of fetus.
- Fetal or maternal infections.
- Multiple pregnancy.

WEIGHT-FOR-GESTATION STANDARDS

- Weight-for-gestation standards are statistical reference levels which enable babies from similar populations to be defined and compared in a uniform manner in terms of weight and gestational age.
- Standard percentile values for birthweight are usually derived from cross-sectional studies and reflect fetal size but *not* fetal growth (see below).
- They need to be established for each population (see Further Reading).

Clinical use of weight-for-gestation standards
- Size (as assessed by weight) at birth is important because when the prognosis for an infant is dependent on the two variables, birthweight and gestational age, birthweight proves to be the more important.
- Most of the infants in whom problems will arise are found in the group weighing less than the tenth percentile for gestational age and sex. These infants are termed 'small-for-dates' (SFD) or 'small-for-gestational-age' (SGA).

Criticisms of weight-for-gestation standards
- Cross-sectional data obtained at birth may not reflect longitudinal fetal growth.
- The weight of babies born at a given gestational age may not be representative of the babies at the same gestational age who remain in utero.
- The charts do not identify those babies whose growth has been retarded but whose birthweight falls above the 10th percentile.
- The charts do not correctly classify those babies who are normally grown but whose weight is below the tenth percentile for gestational age and sex.

Despite these criticisms the tenth percentile cut-off for gestational age and sex for defining SGA infants is useful in clinical practice.

Lowering the percentiles to the fifth or the third is useful in clinical research.

ASSESSMENT OF FETAL STATE

ASSESSMENT OF GESTATIONAL AGE AND/OR FETAL GROWTH

- Menstrual history is an unreliable guide to gestational age in up to 45% of women.
- Serial clinical assessment of *fundal height* (as height in cm above symphysis pubis) provides a guide to fetal growth.
- *Ultrasound: crown–rump (C–R) length*. At 7 weeks menstrual age the C–R length is 10 mm. This has increased to 55 mm by 12 weeks. It provides an accurate estimate of gestational age up to 14 weeks.
- *Ultrasound: bi-parietal diameter (BPD)*. Serial measurements at least 2 weeks apart are widely used to measure fetal growth. When used to indicate fetal maturity it is most accurate before 24 weeks, but unreliable after 28 weeks.
- *Ultrasound: head/abdomen ratio*. Serial ultrasonic measurement (at least 2 weeks apart) of the ratio of the head circumference (at the level of the third ventricle) and the abdominal circumference (at the level of the umbilical vein) is a useful measure of fetal size and growth. The ratio is increased in intrauterine growth retardation (IUGR) because of:
  —sparing of head growth ·
  —reduction in liver size, and therefore abdominal circumference, due to consumption of glycogen reserves.
- *Ultrasound: femur length (FL)*. FL may be a more precise guide to gestational age than BPD. Combining FL and BPD in a predictive formula provides an accurate index of gestational age to 32 weeks.

FETAL WELL-BEING

PRINCIPLES

- The ideal scheme for assessing fetal well-being should:
  —take full account of cycles of normal fetal behaviour
  —detect impending harm accurately (i.e. with high positive and negative predictive powers) and in time to intervene to prevent it
  —give reassurance for as long as possible between tests— preferably up to 7 days
  —avoid causing unnecessary anxiety
  —allow detection of specific causes—e.g. hypoxia, infection, malformations
  —be applicable to large numbers within limited resources
  —produce measurable benefits in reducing perinatal loss or injury—this requires audit of very large numbers of cases.
- Such a system is likely to involve tests which assess several fetal systems (e.g. neurological, cardiovascular and renal), and use

more than one modality (e.g. imaging, cardiotocography, Doppler 'blood flow' studies).
- *The methods should have no known intrinsic risk and observer errors must be minimised by proper training and management.*
- They should be non-obstetrician based, able to be performed rapidly and repeatable sequentially.

FETAL MOVEMENTS

- A daily count of perceived fetal movements from 28 weeks' gestation is a simple and inexpensive routine screening device for monitoring fetal well-being.
- Advice should be sought if fewer than 10 movements are perceived within 12 hours or if the mother feels that 'the baby is not moving'.
- Other tests of fetal welfare can then be applied.

Criticisms of fetal movement counts
- A large number of fetal movements may not be perceived.
- There are great variations in the number of fetal movements from day to day in individual women and from woman to woman.
- The sensitivity and specificity of the method is low.
- One randomised trial suggests a clear benefit, but another does not.
- Less than 1/1000 women might benefit from formal fetal movement counting, using late fetal death as an outcome.
- Formal counting provokes anxiety in about 25% of women. Another 50% are reassured by it.

ANTENATAL FETAL HEART RATE RECORDING

- The 'non-stress test' (NST) is still widely used in the UK as a test of fetal welfare despite lack of evidence of benefit from prospective, properly controlled trials (see CPCD in Further Reading).
- The major hazards are over-interpretation and unnecessary intervention.
- In the clinical setting some reassurance can be obtained from a normal result. The important feature which suggests that the fetus is in good health is the presence of discrete accelerations in response to fetal movements (a 'reactive trace').
- Failure to show reactivity early in the trace is not necessarily abnormal because the fetus has 'rest–activity' cycles and the mean period of rest is about 40 minutes.
- Baseline irregularity is an important feature, but
  —the earlier the gestation the more unreactive the normal trace is
  —the time from 28–32 weeks is a transitional period for the development of baseline irregularity.

- *Decelerations in relation to contractions accompanied by loss of baseline irregularity are a serious prognostic sign.*

BIOPHYSICAL PROFILE (BPP) SCORING

- BPP uses a fetal heart rate (FHR) monitor and a real-time ultrasound machine to assess five 'biophysical' variables:
  —fetal breathing movements
  —discrete body or limb movements
  —fetal tone
  —FHR
  —amniotic fluid volume.
- The technique and interpretation are described in Further Reading.
- BPP scoring does not seem to significantly improve adverse fetal outcome.
- It may, however, still be of value in women at high risk of fetal problems because a normal result is reassuring (but only for up to 24 hours).

DOPPLER STUDIES

The change of frequency of reflected sound from a moving object (Doppler shift) can be used to study non-invasively the movement of blood in vivo. Current systems use the following techniques.

Continuous wave ultrasound
This is the simplest, but movement anywhere along the path of sound is detected.
- It can, therefore, only be used for vessels whose signal pattern (the 'blood velocity waveform') is known.
- *It does not measure flow directly.*
- When the 'blood velocity waveform' is obtained several 'indices' can be measured which depend on the peak systolic (S) and trough diastolic (D) Doppler shifts.
- The three most commonly used are:
  —S/D ratio = S/D
  —resistance index = (S–D)/S
  —pulsatility index = (S–D)/mean.
- A high value for any of these is usually associated with a low blood velocity, which indicates high resistance to flow in the distal vascular bed.
- Since these measurements change with gestation, *results must be compared with appropriate normal ranges.*
- Absent (D=0) or even reverse flow at the end of diastole are strongly suggestive of fetal hypoxia. In the uterine artery waveform, high resistance produces a 'dicrotic' notch, thought to result from failure of trophoblastic invasion of maternal spiral arterioles.

Pulsed-wave systems

Combining this equipment with an imaging ('duplex') system makes studies of utero-placental and fetal vessels more reliable. Since the angle at which the sound hits the vessel (the angle of insonation) is known, blood flow and velocity can be calculated.

Colour flow mapping

The direction of flow is displayed as red or blue depending on whether the blood is moving towards or away from the transducer. Identification of vessels is easier and measurement of the angle of insonation is much easier. This is particularly useful for small vessels (e.g. fetal cerebral circulation).

CLINICAL INDICATIONS FOR DOPPLER STUDIES

- Doppler studies are most useful in the assessment of impaired fetal growth (IUGR) (see below).
- They identify only the sub-group which is hypoxaemic because of inadequate placental function and may be 'abnormal' for up to 18 weeks before any fetal problem is observed.
- They have, as yet, no proven role in population screening for increased risk of pre-eclampsia and/or impaired growth.

INTRAUTERINE GROWTH RETARDATION (IUGR)

- This is *not* synonymous with 'small-for-gestational-age' defined as birthweight less than the tenth (or more rigorously the fifth or third) percentile for gestational age and sex.
- Many infants below the tenth percentile are appropriately grown and healthy.
- Some whose weight lies above the tenth percentile have not achieved their full growth potential and are therefore growth-retarded.

Definition

Failure to achieve full growth potential.

Causes

- Causes of IUGR include:
  —genetic—chromosomal
  —congenital malformations
  —multiple pregnancy
  —chronic maternal or fetal infections
  —maternal smoking
  —factors affecting placental perfusion, e.g. pre-eclampsia, maternal disease processes, high altitude.
- If placental perfusion is impaired, head growth is relatively spared, i.e. IUGR is asymmetrical (see p. 57).

- In the other situations both head and body size are reduced, i.e. IUGR is symmetrical.
- The prognosis for infants with IUGR depends on the aetiology, gestational age and degree of accompanying hypoxia. For neonatal problems see page 174.

FURTHER READING

Chamberlain G (ed) 1995 Turnbull's obstetrics. Churchill Livingstone, Edinburgh

The Cochrane Collaboration 1995 Cochrane Pregnancy and Childbirth Database. BMJ Publishing Group, London

Enkin M, Keirse M J N C, Chalmers I 1989 Effective care in pregnancy and childbirth. Oxford University Press, Oxford

James D K, Steer P J, Weiner C P, Gonik B (eds) 1994 High risk pregnancy—management options. Saunders, London

Rosevear S K, Stirrat G M 1996 Handbook of obstetric management. Blackwell Scientific, Oxford

6. Drugs and pregnancy

DRUGS USED FOR THERAPY

The following are among the factors which must be considered when prescribing any drug during pregnancy and lactation.

- Most drugs, except those with a molecular weight >1000, cross the placenta and are excreted in breast milk.
- The timing of exposure to a 'teratogen' is an important factor in determining the nature and extent of adverse effects.
  - —'Pre-embryonic phase' (days 0–14 after conception)—tends to be an 'all or nothing effect' i.e. damage to all or most cells leads to death: if only a small number of undifferentiated cells are involved, normal development is likely
  - —Embryonic phase (weeks 3–8)—most crucial period for organogenesis and therefore the time of greatest theoretical risk of congenital malformation. Very few drugs, however, have been conclusively shown to be teratogenic
  - —Fetal phase (week 9 to birth)—fetal growth and development can be impaired by drugs taken during this phase. Drugs which cross the placenta may have direct actions on the fetus (e.g. warfarin may cause haemorrhage); some drugs given close to term or during labour may affect the neonate (e.g. diazepam or pethidine).
- Even non-prescription drugs, such as cough medicines (containing iodides), can be harmful; ointments applied to the nipple may be harmful if ingested by the infant.
- Drugs taken by the male partner and excreted in sperm must also be considered, e.g. finasteride for prostatic hypertrophy may be teratogenic to a male fetus; griseofulvin may damage sperm.

PRINCIPLES FOR PRESCRIBING DURING PREGNANCY AND LACTATION

- Drugs should be prescribed for a pregnant woman only when the indications are clear and specific, and the expected benefit to the mother is greater than the risk to the fetus.
- If at all possible, avoid all drugs in the first trimester (even non-prescription drugs).
- Prescribe drugs which have been well tried in pregnancy in preference to newer preparations.

• Use the smallest effective dose for the shortest therapeutic time.

GUIDE TO PRESCRIBING DURING PREGNANCY AND LACTATION

• This can be found in the most current editions of the British National Formulary. See also other suggested titles in Further Reading.
• A National Teratology Information Service has been established to provide information on all aspects of drug use in pregnancy (Telephone: 0191 232 1525).

DRUGS OF ABUSE

Maternal cigarette smoking is associated with an increased risk of low birthweight, microcephaly and facial clefts.

• It is probably the commonest preventable risk marker for late fetal death.
• There is a long-term relation between smoking in pregnancy and the intellectual development of the offspring. These effects are due to
—a direct feto-placental effect of nicotine and its metabolites
—reduced fetal oxygenation.

Alcohol and pregnancy. Excessive chronic alcohol ingestion is usually defined as >80 g/day (equivalent to at least eight large glasses of wine).

• It is associated with a group of fetal problems—the fetal alcohol syndrome. The incidence in North America is between 1 and 2/1000 births. It is less common in the UK despite a high level of alcohol abuse in society.
• The principal features of the fetal alcohol syndrome are: mental retardation, growth retardation and facial anomalies. Other congenital anomalies are also said to be more common.
• The effects of moderate alcohol ingestion (up to 40 g/day) are much more difficult to assess because an accurate drink history is difficult to obtain, and its effects are compounded by other variables such as smoking, social class, age and parity.
• There may be some women in whom the fetus is particularly susceptible to damage from even moderate alcohol ingestion.

Marijuana smoking is associated with a reduction in birthweight. This could be due to:

• the direct effect of cannabis
• reduced fetal oxygenation
• increase in maternal heart rate and blood pressure
• a possible synergistic action with cocaine.

Heroin abuse is associated with an increased risk of pre-term delivery and low birthweight.

- A significant number of newborns have signs of withdrawal—up to 85% if mothers injected heroin, and over 30% for those who smoked it.

Cocaine or 'crack' abuse causes marked vasoconstrictive effects on uteroplacental and fetal vessels.

- This can cause miscarriage, placental abruption, growth retardation, premature delivery, fetal distress and congenital malformations.
- It may affect the neurobehavioural development of the infant and is associated with an increased incidence of sudden infant death.

FURTHER READING

Author anonymous 1996 Pre-conception, pregnancy and prescribing. Drug and Therapeutic Bulletin 4: 25–27

Beeley L, Stirrat G M (eds) 1986 Prescribing in pregnancy. In: Clinics in Obstetrics and Gynaecology 13. Saunders, Eastbourne

British National Formulary 1995 No. 29 et seq. BMA and Pharmaceutical Society of Great Britain, London

Creasy R K, Resnik R (eds) 1994 Maternal–fetal medicine—principles and practice, 3rd edn. Saunders, Philadelphia

Rosevear S K, Stirrat G M 1996 Handbook of obstetric management. Blackwell Scientific, Oxford

Rubin P C 1996 Management of pre-existing disorders in pregnancy: principles of prescribing. Prescribers' Journal 36:21–27

7. Medical and surgical problems in pregnancy

PRE-ECLAMPSIA AND RELATED DISORDERS

Pre-eclampsia (PET) is a disorder of epithelium peculiar to pregnancy which *can affect every system in the body.*
- It is usually characterised by hypertension, renal impairment and fluid retention, and often accompanied by proteinuria and some degree of intravascular coagulation.
- It arises as a consequence of failure of maternal adaptation to pregnancy.
- Although it usually develops in later pregnancy, it occurs as a result of events around implantation.
- It is totally dependent on the presence of trophoblast.
- The pathology begins in the placental bed.

POSTULATED MECHANISM FOR DEVELOPMENT OF PET

Events in early pregnancy
- There is a failure of communication between the conceptus and the mother.
- The mother fails (either totally or partially) to adapt physiologically (see p. 11 for normal adaptive mechanisms).
- Among the consequences may be:
  —trophoblast fails to invade maternal spiral arterioles
  —the predominance of vasodilatory PGI_2 and NO in the endothelium does not occur, so vessels remain responsive to vasoconstrictors
  —maternal plasma volume fails to expand
  —placental bed fails to become a 'low-pressure supply system'.

Prodromal phase
Placental effects
- the placenta is perfused under high pressure
- local endothelial damage causes aggregation of platelets, fibrin and lipid-laden macrophages ('acute atherosis') and micro-thrombi formation
- spiral arterioles become totally or partially occluded
- placental perfusion to the fetus decreases
- placental size is reduced
- endothelial damage begins to extend throughout the maternal vascular tree.

Fetal growth begins to be impaired.

Maternal effects
- vascular resistance (VR) remains high
- cardiac output (CO) is increased
- the physiological fall in blood pressure (VR × CO) does not occur
- at a variable point thereafter, blood pressure begins to rise.

Clinical phase
This classically occurs in the third trimester but it may happen earlier.
- Placental infarction and, sometimes, abruption may occur.
- Pre-eclampsia is the commonest cause of:
  —IUGR in non-malformed infants
  —elective pre-term delivery.
- Perinatal death is increased:
  —in severe disease of early onset (10- to 15-fold)
  —when eclampsia occurs.
- Generalised maternal endothelial damage affects every system in the body with the following maternal effects.

MATERNAL CLINICAL ASPECTS OF PET

The syndrome affects each woman differently. Not all aspects are apparent in each case. Every system can be affected, to a variable and sometimes severe degree.

Cardiovascular and pulmonary effects
- Hypertension (see p. 74) is the commonest manifestation.
- Peripheral oedema occurs due to 'leaky' endothelium.
- Severe pre-eclampsia is a high cardiac output state with inappropriately high systemic vascular resistance. Left ventricular function is hyperdynamic: cardiac failure may supervene in the most severe cases.
- Pulmonary oedema may arise due to an imbalance between a reduced colloid osmotic pressure and the pulmonary capillary wedge pressure. *It can also be precipitated by intravenous fluid overload during treatment without proper monitoring.*
- Acute respiratory distress syndrome (ARDS) caused eight maternal deaths in the UK from 1991–93.

The kidney
- Glomerular endothelial cells swell, blocking the capillaries. (This 'glomerular endotheliosis' is characteristic but not pathognomonic.)
- Impairment of renal function may result in a rise in plasma urate (an early feature), urea and creatinine. Proteinuria (defined as >300 mg/24 h) develops: pre-eclampsia is the commonest cause

of heavy proteinuria in pregnancy and can lead to the nephrotic syndrome.

The liver
Liver involvement must be considered in all cases of severe pre-eclampsia.
- Hepato-cellular damage can occur due to fibrin deposits in the sinusoids.
- Epigastric pain (due to hepatic oedema and distension of the liver capsule) and vomiting are associated with fulminating pre-eclampsia.
- In some cases, jaundice and severe liver damage can follow, often out of proportion to other signs and symptoms.
- The potentially dangerous HELLP syndrome (Haemolysis, Elevated Liver enzymes, and Low Platelets) must be considered in severe cases.
- Subcapsular haemorrhages and even liver rupture may occur.

Coagulation
The physiological changes in the clotting system in pregnancy are outlined on page 14.
- Increasingly generalised endothelial damage commonly causes slight intravascular coagulation, shown by increased platelet turnover and a fall in platelet count (which can be severe in some cases).
- Disseminated intravascular coagulation (DIC) is a rare but serious end point in some cases.
- Haemolysis can occur due to fibrinogen-associated red cell aggregation.

Central nervous system
- Among the signs of CNS involvement are atypical headache, hyperreflexia, visual disturbances and ankle clonus.
- Vasoconstriction of cerebral vessels occurs (probably as a protective mechanism against severe hypertension).
- At a mean arterial pressure of about 130–150 mmHg this mechanism begins to fail, and small vessel walls are damaged and disrupted.
- This can lead to cerebral oedema, haemorrhages and infarcts—all associated with eclampsia (see p. 73), a major cause of maternal death.

MATERNAL MORTALITY AND PRE-ECLAMPSIA/ ECLAMPSIA

'Hypertensive disorders of pregnancy' were the second commonest cause, after thromboembolism, of maternal death in the UK in 1991–93. The number of deaths and percentages of the

Medical and surgical problems in pregnancy

total (see p. 168) from 1985 to 1993 are shown in the information box.

Triennia	Number of deaths			Percentage of total from all causes
	Pre-eclampsia	Eclampsia	Total	
1985–87	15	12	27	19
1988–90	12	14	26	19
1991–93	12	8	20	15.5

Table 7.1 Lists the main causes of deaths in this category.

Table 7.1 Maternal mortality in the UK, 1985–1993

	1985–87	1988–90	1991–93
Cerebral	11	14	5
Intracerebral haemorrhage	11	10	5
Subarachnoid	nil	2	nil
Infarct/oedema	nil	2	nil
Pulmonary	12	10	11
Adult respiratory distress syndrome (ARDS)	9	9	8
Oedema	1	1	3
Haemorrhage	1	nil	nil
Pneumonia	1	nil	nil
Hepatic	1	1	nil
Other	3	2	4

Predisposing factors
- *Primigravidity*. The incidence of severe (proteinuric) pre-eclampsia in a first pregnancy is around 6%.
  —It occurs in about 2% of all second pregnancies, rising to 12% if severe pre-eclampsia (with IUGR) was present in the first, and falling to 0.7% if the first was a singleton, normotensive pregnancy
  —Pregnancy by a new partner may increase the risk to that of a first pregnancy
  —No protection is offered by an early spontaneous or induced abortion.

- *Genetic* It is either due to a dominant gene with varying penetrance or to 'multifactorial' inheritance. Risk is outlined in the information box.

Relative affected	Excess risk in woman being considered
Mother	× 4–5
Sister	× 3–4
Grandmother	× 2–3

—It is also more common when there is a strong family history of hypertension, other cardiovascular disorders or auto-immune disease
—There is no significant racial preponderance.
- *Medical* Among the predisposing factors are pre-existing hypertension, diabetes mellitus, protein S deficiency, activated protein C resistance (see p. 100), anti-cardiolipin antibodies and hyperhomocystinaemia.
- *Socioeconomic* The incidence increases as socioeconomic status deteriorates (associated with poor maternal nutrition?).
—The incidence is lower in women who smoke, but the fetal outlook is poor in smokers who develop pre-eclampsia.
- *Obstetric* Multiple pregnancy and hydatidiform mole are associated with very early and severe pre-eclampsia. It also may occur when hydrops fetalis (Rhesus and non-Rhesus) is present.

PREVENTION OF PRE-ECLAMPSIA

For analysis of clinical trials see Further Reading.

Low-dose aspirin suppresses production of thromboxane A_2 by platelets in vitro without significantly affecting prostacyclin.
—However, the results of published trials do not support routine prophylactic or therapeutic use in women judged to be at added risk of pre-eclampsia or IUGR.
—There may be a small additional risk of ante- or postpartum haemorrhage.
—The only women in whom it may be justified are those with a previous history of early onset pre-eclampsia.

Calcium Randomised controlled trials (RCTs) have, so far, been too small to provide reliable information but calcium supplementation (2 g/day) during pregnancy may reduce the risk of hypertension, pre-eclampsia and pre-term delivery. Larger trials are necessary.

Fish oils It has been suggested their use during pregnancy is associated with a fall in incidence of severe pre-eclampsia and pre-

term delivery. No recommendations can yet be made from
available trials.

MANAGEMENT OF PRE-ECLAMPSIA

The principles are:
- early recognition of the symptomless syndrome
- awareness of serious nature of the condition in its severe form
  without over-reacting to mild disease
- agreed guidelines for admission to hospital, investigation, and
  use of antihypertensive and anticonvulsant therapy
- well-timed delivery to pre-empt serious maternal or fetal complications
- postnatal follow-up and counselling for future pregnancies.

Clinical observation and investigation
Examination (over and above routine):
- palpation of the femoral pulses (to exclude coarctation of aorta)
- look for hyperreflexia and ankle clonus
- check optic fundi for silver wiring, arterio-venous nipping,
  exudates and haemorrhage.

Laboratory investigation
- *Proteinuria*—see page 66. If present also check *urine microscopy
  and culture* to exclude urinary infection.
- *Serum urate* levels increase early in pre-eclampsia. Levels
  >350 µmol/L are abnormal in pregnancy but gradually increasing
  levels are more significant.
- *Serum urea and creatinine*. Rising levels are significant but not
  such sensitive indicators of pre-eclampsia as uric acid. The upper
  limits of normal in pregnancy are 5 mmol/L for serum urea and
  100 µmol/L for creatinine, but trends are even more important
  than specific levels.
- *Platelet count* gradually falls if disseminated intravascular
  coagulation is occurring.
- *Liver function*—this should be checked once persistent
  proteinuria is present, or if platelet count is significantly reduced.
  It can be detected by elevation of liver enzymes (not alkaline
  phosphatase, which is normally raised because it is produced by
  the placenta).
- *Coagulation studies* should be carried out if platelet count is
  reduced, and in severe disease.
- Tests of fetal growth and well-being (see p. 54).
- Each of these tests should be repeated as often as is clinically
  necessary.

Management of mild (non-proteinuric) pre-eclampsia
The principles are:
- uncomplicated hypertension is suitable for careful supervision at
  home by the primary health care team

- the use of sedatives or tranquillisers is contraindicated
- antihypertensive therapy is not indicated (see below)
- admission to hospital is indicated when:
  —SBP is 160 and/or DBP 100 mmHg or greater
  —proteinuria is detected in a clean (i.e. mid-stream) urine sample in the absence of a urinary infection
  —the patient is symptomatic with e.g. visual disturbances, unusual headache, epigastric pain, or vomiting (URGENT!)
  —there is clinical evidence of intrauterine growth retardation
  —tests of fetal welfare have deteriorated (see p. 57)
  —a previous bad obstetric history suggests that closer surveillance would be worthwhile.

MANAGEMENT OF SEVERE HYPERTENSION

- The maternal risks of cerebrovascular accident and of left ventricular or renal failure begin to increase significantly when hypertension is severe.
- The choice has then to be made between delivery and anti-hypertensive therapy.
- Among the factors to be considered are:
  —gestational age—it is seldom justified to commence long-term oral therapy from 34 weeks
  —the severity of other signs and symptoms
  —availability of intensive neonatal care facilities.
- *Treatment neither influences the progression of underlying pre-eclampsia nor significantly improves fetal outcome.* It helps to protect the mother and enables many pregnancies to continue that otherwise would be ended because of maternal risk.

CONTROL OF ACUTE SEVERE HYPERTENSION

- There is no consensus on the optimum acute treatment.
- The important objective is to reduce the blood pressure to safe levels (but not too low!).
- Parenteral *hydralazine* is used most commonly but oral *nifedipine* should be considered (see below). For more detailed discussion see Further Reading.

LONGER-TERM CONTROL OF SEVERE HYPERTENSION
(see Further Reading)

- There is still insufficient trial evidence to determine whether the benefits outweigh any disadvantages.
- If it is to be used, the suggested indications are:
  —DBP ≥100 mmHg
  —pregnancy ≤34 weeks
  —fetal and maternal state otherwise good.
- *Methyldopa* remains the drug of first choice.

- The combined α- and β- blocking agent *labetalol* is commonly used.
- The potent vasodilator and calcium channel blocker *nifedipine* is a useful second-line treatment. Its major drawback is severe headache.
- *Angiotensin-converting enzyme (ACE) inhibitors* have deleterious fetal effects and their use is not recommended. If a woman with chronic hypertension becomes pregnant on an ACE inhibitor, change to another anti-hypertensive agent is advised.

Diuretics
Review of trials does not allow reliable conclusions to be reached. Their use has been discouraged in pre-eclampsia because they further reduce circulating blood volume.

Timing of delivery
- The most common grounds for delivery are:
  —progressive fetal compromise (i.e. when the baby is safer delivered)
  —unacceptable risk to maternal health, e.g. uncontrollable BP, impending renal failure or heart failure, HELLP syndrome, DIC, eclampsia (see below).
- The mode of delivery (caesarean section versus vaginal) depends on:
  —the seriousness of the situation
  —the gestational age
  —the degree of fetal/maternal compromise.
- Epidural analgesia is the method of choice for labour (as long as a coagulation defect has been excluded).
- Appropriate facilities for the care of the newborn infant must be available.

Fluid balance and plasma volume expansion
- Restriction of i.v. fluids to less than 1 litre following delivery of women with severe pre-eclampsia reduces the risk of pulmonary oedema without affecting renal function.
- Diuretics are contraindicated because they aggravate hypovolaemia and can precipitate renal failure.
- Plasma volume expansion accompanied by vasodilator drugs (e.g. hydralazine) may have a role in some severe cases with the following provisos:
  —it must be used only in high-dependency units where invasive monitoring (e.g. to measure pulmonary capillary wedge pressure—PCWP) is available
  —only small volumes (e.g. haemaccel 200–600 ml) are necessary
  —*blind therapy is very dangerous and can lead to pulmonary oedema and death.*
- Central venous pressure (CVP) monitoring may not be adequate. Measurement of PCWP may be required (CVP does not correlate with PCWP when the former is >6 mmHg).

ECLAMPSIA

- Defined as the occurrence of one or more convulsions in association with the syndrome of pre-eclampsia.
- The timing of fits follows: antepartum 38%; intrapartum 18%; postpartum 44%.
- Postpartum fits usually occur within 24 hours of delivery, but rarely occur up to 3 weeks later.
- *Eclampsia is still a major contributor to maternal mortality* (see p. 67).
- In addition to severe hypertension and proteinuria (which may not occur!), among the other symptoms and signs suggesting impending eclampsia are:
  —unusual headache—persistent, severe, generalised (but may be occipital or frontal)
  —visual disturbance—e.g. blurring, flashes or spots, photophobia
  —restlessness, agitation
  —epigastric pain, nausea and vomiting
  —hyperreflexia and clonus
  —retinal oedema, haemorrhages and even papilloedema.

Management
- *Prevention of convulsions*: intravenous and/or intramuscular magnesium sulphate has been used for many years in the USA for the prevention (and treatment) of eclampsia. There is some trial evidence suggesting benefit to both mother and baby (see Further Reading).
- *Control of convulsions*: the Collaborative Eclampsia Trial (see Further Reading) has demonstrated clearly that magnesium sulphate is the drug of choice for treatment of eclampsia. It reduces neuromuscular irritability and causes cerebral depression. The suggested regimes are either:
  —loading dose of 4 g i.v. over 5 minutes
  —followed by 5 g i.m. (into each buttock) and further 5 g i.m. every 4 h

  or

  —i.v. infusion of 1 g/h for 24 h
  —further 2–4 g given i.v. over 5 min if convulsions recur.

  Treatment is monitored clinically by checking respiratory rate (>16/min); urine output (>25 ml/h); and the continuing presence of knee jerks. Serum measurement of magnesium levels is not required.
- *Control of hypertension* (see p. 71).
- *General management*
  —Patency of the airway must be maintained and oxygen given as necessary
  —A urinary catheter should be inserted to monitor urine output

—Check for disorders of electrolyte balance and disseminated intravascular coagulation.
- *Delivery of the infant.* Caesarean section is the method of choice but only when the eclampsia is under control. If eclampsia supervenes when the patient is well advanced in labour, vaginal delivery may be possible.
- ***NSAIDs must be avoided for post-operative analgesia because of the risk of renal failure when used in the presence of severe pre-eclampsia!***

Long-term outlook
- It has for long been thought that severely pre-eclamptic/eclamptic primigravidae are not at increased risk of developing chronic hypertension (given that there is not pre-existing hypertension). There is some evidence that this may not be the case.
- Patients with severe early-onset pre-eclampsia should be screened for protein S and protein C deficiency, activated protein C resistance, anti-cardiolipin antibodies, hyperhomocystinaemia and chronic hypertension because of their increased prevalence in such women.

HYPERTENSION AND RENAL DISEASE

Definitions
Hypertension—two consecutive measurements of diastolic blood pressure (DBP) ≥90 mmHg 4 or more hours apart or one measurement ≥110 mm Hg.
- In the UK the DBP is traditionally taken at the 'point of muffling' (Korotkoff phase IV) in women lying on their side with a 15–30° tilt. In the USA disappearance of the sound (Korotkoff phase V) is used and there is some evidence that this may be more appropriate.
- The use of systolic blood pressure (SBP) or the calculation of mean arterial pressure does not add to the prognostic significance and is more complicated.
- A DBP of 90 mmHg corresponds to the point at which the perinatal mortality rate begins to rise in population studies, and is approximately the mean +3 SD in mid-pregnancy, the mean +2 SD from 34 to 37 weeks, and the mean +1 SD at term. The significance of the same level of hypertension, therefore, varies with the stage in pregnancy at which it is recorded.

Severe hypertension—a DBP ≥120 mmHg on one occasion *or* a DBP ≥110 mmHg on two consecutive occasions 4 or more hours apart.

Proteinuria—a 24-hour urine collection containing ≥300 mg protein. A reagent strip showing 2+ is equivalent to 1 g albumin/L.

Chronic (pre-existing) hypertension
Among the possible causes are:

- essential hypertension—outlook is good in this condition but pre-eclampsia may supervene. Management of the hypertension is as described above
- coarctation of the aorta
- renal hypertension—this is discussed below
- phaeochromocytoma—see page 89.
- auto-immune connective tissue disorders—see page 92
- some drugs, e.g. corticosteroids, MAO (monoamine oxidase) inhibitors.

FURTHER READING

Chamberlain G (ed) 1995 Turnbull's obstetrics. Churchill Livingstone, Edinburgh
The Cochrane Collaboration 1995 Cochrane Pregnancy and Childbirth Database. BMJ Publications, London
Eclampsia Trial Collaborative Group 1995 Which anticonvulsant for women with eclampsia? Evidence from the Collaborative Eclampsia Trial. Lancet 345:1455–1463
James D K, Steer P J, Weiner C P, Gonik B (eds) 1994 High risk pregnancy—management options. Saunders, London
Pijnenborg R 1996 The placental bed. Hypertension in Pregnancy 15(1):7–23
Redman C, Walker I 1992 Pre-eclampsia—the facts. Oxford University Press, Oxford
Rosevear S K, Stirrat G M 1996 Handbook of obstetric management. Blackwell Scientific, Oxford
Teoh T G, Redman C W G 1996 Management of pre-existing disorders in pregnancy: hypertension. Prescribers' Journal 36:28–36

URINARY TRACT INFECTIONS

ASYMPTOMATIC BACTERIURIA

Definition: Cultured urine contains >100 000 organisms/ml.
- Asymptomatic bacteriuria occurs in about 5% of pregnancies.
- *Escherichia coli (E. coli)* is the infecting organism in 90% of cases.
- Pregnancy does not predispose to it but it progresses to acute pyelonephritis in a greater proportion (25–40%) of pregnant women.
- Routine culture of a mid-stream urine (MSU) should be performed at booking because:
  —detection and treatment prevents at least two thirds of the cases of acute pyelonephritis
  —maternal anaemia and IUGR may be more common in untreated cases.
- Recurrent bacteriuria is common.

ACUTE PYELONEPHRITIS

- This usually presents as a febrile illness with loin pain and vomiting.
- It needs to be differentiated from other causes of an acute abdomen.

- It is associated with pre-term labour and, sometimes, fetal death.
- Blood cultures should be taken in severe cases. *E. coli* is the commonest infecting organism.
- Treatment with appropriate antibiotic should begin while urine culture and sensitivity results are awaited. It should continue in full therapeutic doses for 3–6 weeks. Thereafter urine culture should be performed from each antenatal visit.
- If it recurs consider maintenance antibacterial therapy for the remainder of pregnancy and for 2 weeks postpartum.

CHRONIC RENAL DISEASE

- Pregnancy per se does not usually adversely affect most renal diseases, with the possible exception of membrano-proliferative glomerulonephritis and lupus nephropathy.
- The increased risk of urinary infection in pregnancy can lead to exacerbation of chronic pyelonephritis.
- The outcome of pregnancy is proportional to the severity of renal impairment rather than specific diseases.

Pre-pregnancy counselling
- Pregnancy is not advisable in women whose plasma creatinine levels are ≥200 µmol/L and whose DBP is ≥90 mmHg. Most women with severe renal impairment are amenorrhoeic and infertile.
- Among the renal diseases seen in pregnancy are:
  —chronic pyelonephritis—good prognosis if renal function adequate and normotensive
  —chronic glomerulonephritis—patients more liable to develop superadded pre-eclampsia
  —polycystic kidneys—prognosis depends on renal function and level of BP
  —auto-immune connective tissue disease nephropathy—see p. 92
  —diabetic nephropathy—see page 82.

Regular antenatal assessment should be carried out of:
- maternal blood pressure, renal function and urine cultures
- fetal growth and well-being (see p. 54).

NEPHROTIC SYNDROME

Heavy proteinuria (>3.5 g/24 h), with hypoalbuminaemia and gross generalised oedema.
- The commonest cause in late pregnancy is pre-eclampsia.
- If it occurs before 32 weeks' gestation a high-protein diet can be given and salt-free albumin infusions considered after seeking advice from a nephrologist.
- Steroids should not be given unless a biopsy-proven diagnosis

suggests that they would be beneficial (e.g. membrano-proliferative glomerulonephritis).
• Diuretics are contraindicated.

RENAL AND URETERIC CALCULI

If this diagnosis is suspected, intravenous urography is indicated if two of the following are present:
• microscopic haematuria
• recurrent symptoms referable to urinary tract
• sterile urine culture when symptoms suggest pyelonephritis.

Management is initially conservative, with hydration, antibiotics and analgesia. Surgery is rarely necessary.

RENAL ALLOGRAFTS AND PREGNANCY

• Chronic haemodialysis is associated with infertility, and successful pregnancy is uncommon in women receiving this treatment.
• Renal transplantation restores fertility in proportion to reproductive age and allograft function.

Pre-pregnancy counselling
• The following criteria are guides to the timing of pregnancy:
  —at least 18 months since transplant
  —renal function stable, with no proteinuria and plasma creatinine ≤200 µmol/L
  —normotensive (or nearly so)
  —no evidence of graft rejection
  —immunosuppressive therapy at maintenance levels.
• Antenatal care should be hospital-based in a joint clinic involving obstetrician and nephrologist.
• In addition to routine, maternal assessment should include screening for anaemia, any infection, and superadded pre-eclampsia.
• Graft rejection is no more or less common. Renal ultrasonography may be helpful in its detection. Immunosuppressive therapy should be maintained. The effects of cyclosporin therapy in pregnancy need to be evaluated.
• Vaginal delivery should be aimed for. Caesarean section is indicated for obstetric reasons only.
• Fetal outcome is surprisingly good, although pre-term delivery (elective and spontaneous) and IUGR are more common. Congenital malformations are not more common. Neonates may be more prone to viral or other infections.

There is disagreement as to whether breast-feeding is or is not to be encouraged.
    Postpartum contraception poses a problem. On balance, a low-

dose combined pill (see p. 214) may be best as long as surveillance is frequent.

FURTHER READING

Chamberlain G (ed) 1995 Turnbull's obstetrics. Churchill Livingstone, Edinburgh
James D K, Steer P J, Weiner C P, Gonik B (eds) 1994 High risk pregnancy—
    management options. Saunders, London

ANAEMIA

- The haemoglobin (Hb) concentration falls during pregnancy (but not normally below 10.4 g/dl) because the physiological increase in plasma volume outstrips that of the red cell mass.
- The average requirement for iron is about 4 mg/day, increasing as the pregnancy progresses. Although the normal diet contains up to 25 mg/day of iron only about 10% of this is absorbed. Iron stores fall, therefore, during pregnancy. The first effect is a fall in serum ferritin to around 6 µg/L by 28 weeks. Hb does not fall, and microcytic erythrocytes do not appear for several weeks after the stores are exhausted.
- At present trial data do not recommend routine supplementation with iron and folate of all pregnant women in well-nourished communities.

IRON DEFICIENCY

The blood film is hypochromic and microcytic. Mean corpuscular haemoglobin (MCH) is decreased; serum ferritin levels are low (<15 µg/L) and iron-binding capacity is increased.

Treatment

- Increase dietary sources of iron (e.g. meat, fish, eggs and spinach) and supplement with oral iron. If gastrointestinal intolerance to iron occurs, change to a chelated or delayed-release preparation. Parenteral iron is rarely necessary.
- An underlying folate deficiency may be unmasked by treatment.

FOLATE DEFICIENCY

Blood film is normochromic and macrocytic. Red cells may be nucleated and contain Howell–Jolly nuclear inclusion bodies.
- Check serum folate and B_{12} (red cell folate is low in both folate and B_{12} deficiency and is therefore not so helpful).

Treatment

Increase dietary sources of folate (as for iron). Give 5–15 mg folic acid orally daily.

VITAMIN B$_{12}$ DEFICIENCY

- Vitamin B$_{12}$ deficiency is rare in pregnancy, with a higher incidence in strict vegetarians. Blood film is megaloblastic.
- Treatment is with intramuscular vitamin B$_{12}$. A daily folate supplement of 300 µg will not mask vitamin B$_{12}$ deficiency.

SICKLE CELL DISEASE

- For genetics see page 43
- Major problem is Hb S/S, with Hb S/C and Hb S/Thal being less common
- Perinatal loss and IUGR are common.

Antenatal screening Routine Hb electrophoresis is indicated when the indigenous or immigrant population makes the risk of haemoglobinopathy high.

Sickling crises Hb A and its abnormal variants function similarly when well-oxygenated but the latter polymerise when deoxygenated. The red cells become sickle-shaped and occlude vessels, causing widespread vascular damage, severe pain and haemolytic anaemia.

Prevention Folate supplements and oral bicarbonate (to increase the pH of the urine); blood transfusion (3–4 units) at 6-week intervals; prompt treatment of infection.

SICKLE CELL TRAIT (Hb A/S)

This is usually benign, but sickling cases occur under extreme hypoxia. The Hb level tends to be lower than average. It may predispose to pyelonephritis.

MANAGEMENT OF SEVERE ANAEMIA IN PREGNANCY

- If Hb is <6.0 g/dl then consider exchange transfusion or plasmaphoresis.
- If Hb is between 6.0 and 8.0 g/dl then transfuse slowly with 3–5 units of packed cells. Use intravenous frusemide 20 mg to prevent circulatory overload.

CARDIAC DISEASE

The haemodynamic changes which occur during pregnancy (see p. 12) impose an increased burden on the mother's heart. This causes no problems for healthy women but may do so in women with cardiac disease.

RHEUMATIC HEART DISEASE (RHD)

- The incidence of RHD has decreased dramatically over the past 25 years in most developed countries.
- Mitral stenosis is still the commonest and most important problem.
- Pregnancy has no permanent deleterious effect on RHD.

CONGENITAL HEART DEFECTS (CHD)

- An increasing number of women with CHD are reaching childbearing age as a result of improved medical and surgical management.
- Most women with acyanotic CHD tolerate pregnancy well (except those with severe aortic stenosis and coarctation of the aorta).
- Patients with uncorrected CHD, pulmonary hypertension (either primary or as part of Eisenmenger's syndrome) do badly, and maternal death can occur suddenly.

OTHER CARDIAC LESIONS

- Tachyarrhythmias—see below
- Myocardial infarction—a rare complication of pregnancy; risk factors include smoking, hypertension, diabetes mellitus and familial hypercholesterolaemia.

PRE-CONCEPTION COUNSELLING

This is important for women with known heart disease because:
- treatment can be made optimal
- a specific plan can be prepared for pregnancy
- surgery can be advised in those women in whom pregnancy would add a severe but correctable burden, e.g. tight mitral stenosis
- advice can be given to those women at high risk during pregnancy, e.g. Marfan's syndrome, inoperable cyanotic heart disease, primary pulmonary hypertension, Eisenmenger's syndrome; *pregnancy may be best avoided in these conditions*.

ANTENATAL MANAGEMENT

Termination of pregnancy is not medically indicated, except when pulmonary hypertension is severe.
- Arrange regular antenatal visits to obstetrician and cardiologist.
- Ensure adequate rest.
- Stongly advise against smoking.
- Prevent anaemia.
- Treat respiratory infection promptly.
- Cover dental work with antibiotics.

- Be watchful for incipient pulmonary congestion and arrhythmias.

MANAGEMENT OF LABOUR

- Aim for vaginal delivery at term. Induction of labour is necessary only for obstetric reasons. Vaginal prostaglandins are the method of choice because early amniotomy may increase the risk of infection.
- When patient starts labour with good cardiac reserve the risk of heart failure is low.
- Cover labour with antibiotics.
- Control any infusion of parenteral fluids very strictly.
- Provide adequate analgesia—epidural anaesthesia is safe in *experienced* hands as long as hypotension is avoided; it is contraindicated in hypertrophic obstructive cardiomyopathy (HOCM) (see below) and Eisenmenger's syndrome.
- Avoid aortocaval compression.
- Shorten the second stage by use of 'lift-out' forceps or vacuum extractor (without raising legs into lithotomy position if possible).
- Ergometrine is best avoided.
- Do not attempt caesarean section in the presence of heart failure.
- Have oxygen and relevant drugs *immediately available*.
- Avoid β-sympathomimetic drugs in women with pre-existing heart disease.

SPECIFIC PROBLEMS

CARDIAC FAILURE

- The principles of diagnosis and treatment are the same as in the non-pregnant patient.
- It can occur even in young asymptomatic women with cardiac disease at any stage of pregnancy.
- Sudden cardiac decompensation is more likely to occur shortly after delivery.

ACUTE PULMONARY OEDEMA

A medical emergency which demands immediate attention.

Management

- Nurse in semi-recumbent position, give oxygen and keep airways clear.
- Give intravenous morphine, aminophylline, frusemide and digoxin (if not previously digitalised). In labour the fetus must take second place until the situation is under control.

TACHYARRHYTHMIAS

Atrial fibrillation is a medical emergency requiring bed rest in hospital and digitalisation. The advice of a cardiologist must always be sought. Anticoagulation may also be indicated.

Atrial tachycardia can precipitate heart failure rapidly. It often responds to carotid sinus pressure.

CARDIAC SURGERY AND PREGNANCY

- Anticoagulant therapy must be maintained and carefully controlled in women who have had previous cardiac surgery.
- Warfarin is the drug of choice here even in the first trimester. Intravenous heparin should be substituted 2–3 weeks before anticipated time of delivery (see p. 101).
- Mitral valvotomy may be indicated during pregnancy in pure severe mitral stenosis if pulmonary congestion develops, or if there is no prompt response to medical therapy.

HYPERTROPHIC OBSTRUCTIVE CARDIOMYOPATHY (HOCM)

- Most women with HOCM tolerate pregnancy and vaginal delivery well. This depends, however, on the severity of the left ventricular outflow tract obstruction.
- It is important to avoid:
  —digoxin therapy
  —β-sympathomimetic drugs—some of the deaths associated with their use have been in women with undiagnosed cardiomyopathy
  —aortocaval compression—e.g. the left lateral position should be used for delivery.
- Caesarean section should be reserved for obstetric indications.

DIABETES MELLITUS (DM)

Definition

Fasting venous plasma glucose concentration ≥8.0 mmol/L *and* ≥11.0 mmol/L 2 hours after a 75 g oral glucose load; *or* one of these plus symptoms and signs (polydipsia, polyuria, weight loss).

Impaired glucose tolerance (IGT) is present if the fasting level is <8.0 mmol/L but rises to 8.0–10.9 mmol/L 2 hours after 75 g oral glucose load.

ANTENATAL SCREENING

IGT/DM must be suspected in all women with:
- significant glycosuria on two occasions antenatally or in a single fasting urine sample

- mother, father or siblings with diabetes
- previous babies >90th percentile for gestational age and sex
- diabetes in a previous pregnancy
- previous unexpected perinatal death
- polyhydramnios
- maternal obesity (>20% above ideal weight).

Routine antenatal screening has been recommended because:
- about 30% of gestational diabetes patients have none of the above risk features
- not all women with IGT or even diabetes have persistent glycosuria
- glycosuria can be found in the urine of up to 50% of all pregnant women at some time.

Selective or comprehensive screening can be undertaken by:
- random blood glucose estimations at booking and at 28–32 weeks. Further investigation is required for levels ≥6.4 mmol/L within 2 hours of the last meal or ≥5.8 mmol/L more than 2 hours after it
- estimation of blood glucose concentrations fasting and 2 hours after a 50 g glucose load. An oral 75 g glucose tolerance test (GTT) is indicated if fasting and/or the 2-hour levels exceed 5 and 7 mmol/L respectively.

RISKS ASSOCIATED WITH DIABETES

All risks are increased by poor control of diabetes (especially if keto-acidosis develops) and by inadequate obstetric supervision.
- Maternal—retinopathy, nephropathy and neuropathy may be worsened
- Congenital malformations—there is a slight general increase in malformations related to hyperglycaemia during organogenesis, especially craniospinal and cardiac defects; sacral agenesis is a rare anomaly specifically associated with diabetes
- Obstetric complications—e.g. polyhydramnios, pre-term labour, pre-eclampsia
- Infections—urinary, monilial and other infections
- Sudden unexpected fetal death (SUFD)—increased risk during the last 4–6 weeks of pregnancy
- Difficult delivery—because of excess fetal growth (macrosomia)
- Neonatal problems—birth trauma, hyaline membrane disease, hypoglycaemia, hypomagnesaemia, hypocalcaemia, jaundice.

Macrosomia has been reported in up to 30% of seemingly well-controlled diabetics.

MANAGEMENT

Pre-pregnancy counselling allows:
- general advice, e.g. about tight diabetic control (particularly around conception and in the early weeks of pregnancy)

- planning for pregnancy (including early booking for antenatal care)
- review of diet
- examination of optic fundi
- establishment of good blood glucose control.

Antenatal care for pre-existing diabetics should be jointly between obstetrician and physician. For optimal *diabetic* control:
- organise high-fibre diet with correct calorific intake and CHO content
- carry out blood glucose profiles two or three times/week at home using filter-paper strips or a reflectance meter. Tests are carried out before and 2 hours after each meal and last thing at night. Pre- and post-prandial levels of <5.0 and <7.0 mmol/L respectively are ideal
- regular urinalysis (mainly to check on carbohydrate loss)
- regular glycosylated haemoglobin or fructosamine estimations (mainly to provide retrospective information on the validity of home glucose monitoring)
- *insulin treatment* is best using combined soluble and intermediate-acting insulins morning and evening or intermittent soluble insulin with each meal (three times a day) and an intermediate acting insulin in the evening. Human or highly purified porcine insulins reduce the risk of developing antibodies (which can cross the placenta)
- *maternal health* is also monitored carefully, paying particular attention to weight, optic fundi, blood pressure, and renal function
- *fetal welfare* should be monitored carefully:
  —Carry out baseline scans to confirm gestational age and, at 20 weeks', to exclude major anomalies (especially cranio-spinal and cardiac defects)
  —Continue with serial scans for reduced and, particularly, excess fetal growth
  —Assess fetal well-being (see p. 57) regularly from 28 weeks
  —If macrosomia arises check ultrasound scans for fetal cardiac enlargement.

Admission to hospital is indicated if:
- good glucose control cannot be achieved as an outpatient
- severe hypertension or pre-eclampsia develop
- weight gain is excessive
- renal function deteriorates
- fetal well-being causes concern.

Gestational diabetes
- If IGT is discovered during pregnancy, carry out blood glucose profile (as above).
- Treatment is indicated for glucose levels ≥5.8 mmol/L.

- Dietary control should be attempted initially. If this is not successful then insulin should be prescribed. Management is then as above for established diabetes.

Labour and delivery
- When diabetes is well controlled and *pregnancy is uncomplicated* vaginal delivery between 38 and 40 weeks should be anticipated.
  - —During labour close control of blood glucose is achieved by a continuous infusion of soluble insulin (usually 50 units in 50 ml normal saline), and a separate infusion of 5% dextrose with KCl (10 mmol in 500 ml) added. The dextrose and KCl infusion should run at a constant rate (100 ml/h)
  - —Regular blood glucose monitoring should be undertaken and the insulin infusion titrated to keep levels between 5 and 7 mmol/L
  - —If a syntocinon infusion is necessary this should be made up using normal saline
  - —Continuous electronic fetal monitoring is advised.
- If elective caesarean section is planned, careful control is necessary before, during and afterwards until the woman can eat and drink normally.
- If pre-term labour supervenes, β-sympathomimetics and steroids are best avoided but, if absolutely necessary, can be covered by appropriate insulin infusions.

Postnatal care
- Insulin sensitivity increases immediately after delivery of the placenta. The required dose of insulin therefore falls quickly and careful monitoring is necessary.
- Hypoglycaemia is common in the neonate and must be treated promptly.
- Breast-feeding is to be encouraged.

Perinatal mortality among diabetic women is now approaching that for other pregnancies (once congenital malformations are excluded), in the best centres.

OTHER ENDOCRINE PROBLEMS

PITUITARY

Prolactin secretion increases from the anterior pituitary throughout pregnancy in response to oestrogen stimulation. By term the concentration has increased ten- to twenty-fold. Basal concentrations fall rapidly after delivery but remain above the normal range in lactating women. Suckling induces a prompt release and levels rise five- to ten-fold. Its main role in pregnancy is trophic action on the breast. After delivery it initiates and maintains lactation, and prevents ovulation (a contraceptive function).

Prolactinoma
Expansion of a prolactinoma is unusual during pregnancy. Conservative management is usually appropriate.
- If being treated with bromocriptine—stop it as soon as pregnancy is diagnosed.
- Check visual fields at 6-week intervals.
- If severe headaches develop or visual fields become impaired, admit to hospital. If fetal maturity allows, deliver, probably by caesarean section. As oestrogen levels fall the prolactin level and volume of the prolactinoma will fall. If the fetus is too immature give bromocriptine 5 mg daily, doubling each day to 20 mg/day in divided doses or until side-effects prevent further increase.
- If visual fields continue to deteriorate add dexamethasone to reduce intracranial swelling, and deliver by caesarean section within 48 hours.
- Breast-feeding is not contraindicated in the presence of a prolactinoma.

THYROID

The main physiological changes in pregnancy are:
- renal clearance of iodide doubles in the first trimester and then remains stable. The result is a low plasma iodide. This is only significant when dietary iodine intake is inadequate, when goitre can develop
- the level of thyroid-binding proteins (globulin, pre-albumin and albumin) more than doubles due to an oestrogen effect on the liver. Although total T_3 and T_4 levels rise markedly, the levels of free hormones fall gradually (but remain within normal limits) as pregnancy progresses
- basal metabolic rate (BMR) increases by up to 30% by the third trimester. This is necessary because of the requirements of the uterus and fetus (75% of the change) and increased maternal respiratory and cardiac effort (25% of the change)
- thyroid-stimulating hormone (TSH) levels are unchanged in pregnancy
- the pregnant woman is basically euthyroid.

HYPERTHYROIDISM

- Complicates 2/1000 pregnancies but has usually been diagnosed and treated before pregnancy.
- The main cause is Graves' disease, but toxic multinodular or solitary nodular goitre may occur. Solitary nodules require careful evaluation because of the risk of malignancy. Fine-needle aspiration is appropriate.

- Uncontrolled hyperthyroidism is associated with increased risk of IUGR, pre-term labour and fetal and neonatal death. The most frequent cause is an auto-antibody which crosses the placenta. It may cause neonatal hyperthyroidism, which has a high mortality rate (up to 25% of cases).

Signs and symptoms
The symptoms overlap with those of normal pregnancy, and palpable thyroid enlargement may be physiological in pregnancy. Biochemical diagnosis is essential.

Diagnosis Free T_3 raised; free T_4 raised or normal; TSH suppressed.

Treatment Carbimazole or propylthiouracil with thyroxine supplement.
- These drugs cross the placenta and can therefore affect the fetal thyroid. However, the balance of risk is in their favour. When control is achieved the drugs can be reduced gradually.
- Propranolol may be used to control serious peripheral effects of thyrotoxicosis.
- Breast-feeding is not necessarily contraindicated.
- Sub-total thyroidectomy may be indicated if a large goitre is causing obstruction, drugs fail to control the symptoms, or there are toxic reactions to drugs.
- Babies born to thyrotoxic mothers should be screened for hypothyroidism.

HYPOTHYROIDISM
- The main causes of primary hypothyroidism are idiopathic, Hashimoto's thyroiditis and post-ablative.
- Treated hypothyroidism due to auto-immune disease or following partial thyroidectomy is not uncommon (about 9/1000 pregnancies).
- Untreated hypothyroidism in early pregnancy has a high fetal wastage or can lead to mental retardation, deafness and cerebral palsy. Later in pregnancy cretinism results.
- Myxoedema rarely presents in pregnancy because sufferers tend to be infertile.

Signs and symptoms
Cold intolerance, changes in skin or hair texture, delayed reflexes, bradycardia. A goitre may be present.

Diagnosis Free T_4 reduced; TSH high. These can also be used to test adequacy of replacement therapy.

Treatment Thyroxine replacement.

- Breast-feeding is not contraindicated.
- If mother has previously had thyrotoxicosis, check for neonatal thyrotoxicosis. If she has had auto-immune thyroiditis, check baby for hypothyroidism.

POSTPARTUM THYROIDITIS

- This is said to occur in 5–9% of pregnancies and is generally unrecognised.
- It presents with fatigue, palpitations or other features of mild hyperthyroidism 2–4 months postpartum, and is often confused with 'postpartum blues'.
- It is commonly associated with HLA DR3, 4 or 5.
- Up to 25% of affected women will have a first-degree relative with a history of thyroid disease. Such women should be screened for thyroid antibodies at booking.

Diagnosis T_3 and T_4 levels are raised. Radioactive iodine uptake is low. Thyroid antimicrosomal antibodies are present.

Treatment Postpartum thyroiditis is usually a self-limiting condition, but hypothyroidism may persist in a small minority. In the thyrotoxic phase β-blocking agents may be used. In the hypothyroid phase thyroxine can be given for 4–6 months.

ADRENAL CORTEX

Among the physiological changes which occur in pregnancy are:
- aldosterone levels rise within days of conception due to an increase in angiotensin II. This reaction is necessary in pregnancy to conserve sodium
- plasma cortisol levels, both bound and free, are elevated with loss of the normal diurnal variation. This increase is due to a slight rise in ACTH as a result of placental secretion
- deoxycorticosterone (DOC) shows the largest increase of all adrenal steroids, starting by 8 weeks' gestation. DOC is not suppressible by dexamethasone during pregnancy. It may be intimately involved with parturition
- plasma testosterone rises secondary to the rise in sex hormone-binding globulin, although it is likely that unbound testosterone is unchanged.

ADDISON'S DISEASE (PRIMARY HYPOADRENALISM)

- This is a rare complication of pregnancy.
- If diagnosed and treated before pregnancy, corticosteroid therapy must continue.
- Additional supplementation will be necessary at times of stress (e.g. labour) or if any infection occurs.

CUSHING'S SYNDROME

- This is a rare but serious condition in pregnancy.
- Fetal loss is common and there is a significant risk to the mother's life.
- The main causes are pituitary adenoma, and adrenocortical adenoma or carcinoma.
- The presentation is as in the non-pregnant.

ADRENAL MEDULLA—PHAEOCHROMOCYTOMA

- The catecholamines adrenaline and noradrenaline do not change in pregnancy.
- This tumour rarely complicates pregnancy, but the consequences for the mother are serious if it goes undetected. Only about half the cases are diagnosed antenatally.
- Patients may present with sustained or paroxysmal hypertension. The other classical symptoms of headache, palpitations and excess sweating may not occur in pregnancy.
- It can cause sudden collapse in pregnancy, labour or the puerperium.
- It should be excluded:
  —when severe or intermittent hypertension occurs (particularly in early pregnancy)
  —in the presence of above 'classical' symptoms
  —in women with a family history of phaeochromocytoma or associated syndromes, e.g. neurofibromatosis or multiple endocrine neoplasia.

Diagnosis Estimation of catecholamines in a properly collected 24-hour urine sample. Ultrasound may detect a suprarenal mass. CT scan or MRI are useful for further localisation.

Treatment α-adrenergic blockade using phenoxybenzamine.
- Control may take 10–14 days.
- Beta adrenergic blockade using propanolol may be necessary to treat tachyarrhythmias. α-blockade must be achieved first.
- Before 23 weeks' gestation the tumour should be removed. From 24 weeks' gestation the pregnant uterus makes this technically difficult. Surgical removal can be delayed until fetal maturity is adequate as long as α-blockade is achieved.
- Removal should be considered with elective caesarean section. Specialist anaesthesia is required, and initial postoperative management must be in an intensive care unit.

IMMUNOLOGICAL DISORDERS

For a description of the immune system and its function see Further Reading.

The major factors protecting the semi-allogeneic (foreign) fetus and placenta from maternal immune attack are:
- the absence of class I (HLA A,B,C) and class II (HLA DP, DQ, DR) major histocompatibility complex (MHC) antigens from villous trophoblast
- the presence on extravillous trophoblast of non-classical MHC antigens to which T cells cannot respond
- protective responses may occur to minor trophoblast antigens
- local immune response may be suppressed by non-specific suppressor cells and other factors in the maternal decidua.

The placenta acts as a barrier to the passage of maternal cells to the fetus. IgG, but not IgM, is actively transported. This provides passive immunity to the fetus but can also cause pathology, e.g. Rhesus haemolytic disease, and allo-immune thrombocytopenia.

IMMUNE THROMBOCYTOPENIA

Platelet mass and turnover increase in pregnancy. The count may fall slightly in normal pregnancy. Thrombocytopenia is defined as a platelet count below $100 \times 10^9 \, l^{-1}$ but major clinical concern arises at counts around $50 \times 10^9 \, l^{-1}$.

Auto-immune (or idiopathic) thrombocytopenia (ITP)
Affects about 1/1000 pregnancies.
- IgG antiplatelet auto-antibodies bind to platelet-specific antigens and cause them to be sequestered in the spleen.
- ITP occurs more commonly in women than in men, with a peak incidence at the height of the reproductive years.

Maternal risks have been overstated. The major hazard is postpartum haemorrhage with an incidence of over 30% if platelet count is below $100 \times 10^9 \, l^{-1}$.

Fetal risk
- The IgG antiplatelet antibodies cross the placenta, but maternal platelet count is a poor predictor of fetal/neonatal thrombocytopenia.
- The principal fetal risk is *intracranial haemorrhage (ICH)* but this has been overstated.
- There is no evidence that elective caesarean section reduces the risk, but it is indicated in the pre-term infant and for breech presentation.

Investigation of mother with ITP
- If platelet count $\geq 100 \times 10^9 \, l^{-1}$ check it at booking, 28 and 34 weeks, and at onset of labour.
- If count $< 50 \times 10^9 \, l^{-1}$, or if there is haemorrhage, exclude other causes—e.g. clotting disorder, pre-eclampsia. The value of measuring platelet auto-antibodies is not proven.

Investigation of fetus
- *Antenatal ultrasound* can help to exclude ICH in utero.
- *Fetal scalp sampling* in labour is not helpful.
- *Cordocentesis* will give an accurate picture of the fetal state but its morbidity does not justify its use except under exceptional circumstances.

Treatment
- *Corticosteroids*—if maternal platelet count <50 × 10^9 l^{-1}.
- *Immunoglobulin* infusion is best restricted to steroid-resistant cases.
- *Platelet transfusions* give only short-lived benefit. They can be used to cover delivery if platelet count is <30 × 10^9 l^{-1}.
- *Plasmaphoresis* may be used when other medical management has failed.
- Any woman who has had a splenectomy should take daily oral penicillin for life to protect against pneumococcal infections. A normal platelet count in a woman who has had a splenectomy does not mean that the fetus will be unaffected.

Feto-maternal allo-immune thrombocytopenia (FMAITP)
FMAITP is analogous to Rhesus disease.
- The incidence may be as high as 1–2/1000 pregnancies.
- The majority of cases in a Caucasian population are due to antibodies against the platelet antigens HPA-1a (75%) or HPA-5b (20%). The remainder are due to antibodies against other antigens (HPA-1 to HPA-9).
- Maternal platelets are normal but the fetus is at significant risk of intracranial haemorrhage.
- The first pregnancy is affected in up to 50% of cases, as are almost 100% of subsequent pregnancies in which the fetus is antigen-positive.
- Routine screening for maternal anti-platelet antibodies during pregnancy is currently only at the trial stage.
- If FMAITP is suspected or has been confirmed in a previous pregnancy:
  —check maternal serum for anti-platelet antibodies
  —determine maternal and paternal HPA status if not already known.
- Fetal HPA status can be ascertained by cell culture from *amniocentesis* or from fetal lymphocytes or platelets obtained by *cordocentesis* (see p. 51).
- The fetal platelet count can also be determined by cordocentesis and fetal immunoglobulin or platelets can be given if required.
- Elective caesarean section is indicated if the fetal platelet count is <50 × 10^9 l^{-1}.

Feto-maternal allo-immune neutropenia (FAN)
- This is the neutrophil equivalent of FMAITP which also can affect first pregnancies.

- The incidence is 0.5–1/1000 livebirths.
- Its clinical significance relates to the infant's ability to combat infection.
- Investigation is as above. Cordocentesis is more difficult to justify because of the less favourable fetal risk/benefit ratio as compared to FMAITP.

SYSTEMIC LUPUS ERYTHEMATOSUS (SLE)

A multisystem disease of unknown aetiology that tends to occur in women of reproductive age.
- The diagnosis rests on the presence of criteria suggested by the American Rheumatism Association (see Tan et al, in Further Reading). The most helpful serological tests are anti-nuclear factor and anti-DNA antibodies.
- Pregnancy has no specific effects on SLE except for an increased risk of exacerbation during the puerperium.
- Women with SLE in pregnancy have an increased risk of:
  —first-trimester pregnancy loss
  —lupus nephritis
  —hypertension in pregnancy
  —transient neonatal SLE—permanent congenital heart block may occur in association with anti-Ro antibodies.
- A seemingly healthy woman delivering a baby with CHB should be observed for the development of SLE.

Management during pregnancy
- Close antenatal supervision is necessary, with particular attention to serial measurements of blood pressure, renal function and fetal growth.
- The mainstay of treatment is maternal corticosteroid therapy but azathioprine may be needed in some circumstances.
- The timing of delivery depends on the severity of the condition, and deteriorating renal function may be an indication for early delivery.
- If the fetus has congenital heart block then caesarean section is warranted.

Lupus anticoagulant (LA) or inhibitor is a circulating anti-cardiolipin antibody which acts on the clotting cascade.
- All phospholipid-dependent coagulation tests, e.g. activated partial thromboplastin time (APTT) and kaolin clotting time (KCT), tend to be prolonged even after the addition of normal plasma.
- It is associated with a high prevalence of maternal thrombosis and fetal loss.
- It is not specific to SLE and may be found in any woman with a history of unexplained fetal loss at any gestational age.
- Corticosteroids and low-dose aspirin have been used successfully to treat affected women.

MYASTHENIA GRAVIS

A rare auto-immune condition with a peak incidence between 20 and 30 years of age frequently associated with a thymoma or thymic lymphoid hyperplasia.

- It produces rapid fatigue and weakness of voluntary muscles.
- Pregnancy does not worsen the disease but exacerbations can occur (most frequently in the puerperium) in up to 30% of women.
- The antibody can cross the placenta and cause a transient (or rarely permanent) effect on fetal voluntary muscles.
- Among the drugs which can exacerbate it are sedatives, tranquillisers, analgesics and narcotics.
- Treatment is with anticholinesterase drugs such as neostigmine (with atropine) or pyridostigmine. Corticosteroids or ACTH may also be effective.
- Labour may be shorter than usual but the effort of the second stage can be tiring. Elective forceps delivery is usually indicated.
- General anaesthesia requiring muscle relaxation can result in prolonged paralysis of voluntary muscles.

RHESUS ISO-IMMUNISATION

THE RH FACTOR

Each Rh gene is made up of three components from three allelomorphic pairs—C or D or d, E or e. Each parent passes on either the first or second half of his/her full genotype, e.g. CDe/cde parents hand on their CDe or cde.

All Rh-negative people have 'd' in each half of the genotype. Where 'D' occurs in both halves of the genotype a parent is homozygous and passes on only the Rh-D-positive gene.

Clinically significant rhesus iso-immunisation is usually against the D antigen. Anti-c or anti-Kell antibodies may also cause problems.

SENSITISATION

- Sensitisation may occur antenatally in 1–2% of previously unsensitised Rh-D-negative women in the absence of any overt complications.
- It usually occurs at parturition due to feto-maternal haemorrhage.
- Other causes of transplacental haemorrhage include abortion (spontaneous or induced), abruptio placentae, amniocentesis and external cephalic version.

PREVENTION

- Anti-D immunoglobulin 500 i.u. (100 µg) can eliminate up to 4.0 ml of Rh-D-positive blood from the maternal circulation.

- It should be given in this dose to all Rh-D-negative women within 60 hours of delivering a Rh-D-positive infant from 20 weeks' gestation (or after a severe placental abruption). If a Kleihauer test demonstrates a feto-maternal transfusion (FMT) of >4.0 ml, additional anti-D must be given.
- 250 i.u. (50 µg) should be given to Rh-D-negative women as soon as possible after a potentially sensitising event. Any FMT >2.0 ml requires additional anti-D.
- Anti-D 500 i.u. at 28 and 34 weeks should be given to Rh-D-negative primigravidae and other previously unsensitised women. This would reduce the incidence of Rh sensitisation by at least a factor of 8.
- The continued occurrence of Rh iso-immunisation is due to failure to give any or enough anti-D when indicated.

DETECTION

In unsensitised women check for Rh antibodies at booking, 28, 32 and 36 weeks.

PREDICTION OF SEVERITY

Obstetric history
- It tends to become more severe in successive pregnancies.
- If at least one child has died from Rhesus haemolytic disease the chance of this pregnancy ending successfully is less than 50%.

Paternal genotype
- About 75% of the fathers of affected children are homozygous (R_1R_1).

Maternal antibody levels
- Once antibodies are detected they must be measured at least monthly thereafter.
- Serum antibody protein levels are of greater predictive value than antibody titres.
- A rapid increase suggests that acute haemolysis will be occurring in the fetus, and amniotic fluid analysis is necessary.

Amniotic fluid analysis
- Maternal IgG crosses the placenta and will cause a fetal haemolytic anaemia.
- Amniotic fluid bilirubin concentrations correlate well with the severity of the haemolysis.
- Spectrophotometry at an optical density (OD) of 450 nm shows a peak directly proportional to the quantity of bilirubin.
- If a previous pregnancy has been complicated by Rh-iso-immunisation, the first amniocentesis should be 10 weeks before the earliest previous intrauterine transfusion, intrauterine death or delivery of a fatally or severely affected infant, but not

before 20 weeks' gestation.
- The second should be 3–4 weeks later. The necessity for, and interval between, subsequent amniocenteses are determined by bilirubin levels.

Fetal blood sampling
- Fetal blood sampling under ultrasound guidance can be used to check fetal haematocrit.
- It is indicated in patients at risk of severe early disease or if amniotic fluid analysis in later second and third trimesters suggests that the baby is severely affected.

INTRAUTERINE TRANSFUSION

- If the fetus is severely affected between 24 and 31 weeks' gestation, direct intravascular fetal blood transfusion (IVT) can be carried out under ultrasound guidance; transfusions can be repeated fortnightly.
- It is particularly useful if hydrops is present, but should be carried out only in specialised centres.
- Intraperitoneal transfusion can be used in conjunction with IVT in the absence of hydrops.

TESTING THE BABY AT BIRTH

Cord blood is taken routinely from the babies of all Rh-D-negative mothers for Hb and film, Coombs' test and bilirubin levels.

RESPIRATORY DISEASES
BRONCHIAL ASTHMA

- Pregnancy has no consistent effect on asthma, and cases should be managed medically in the normal manner using sympathomimetic bronchodilators (e.g. salbutamol or orciprenaline) or disodium cromoglycate.
- If steroids are used, or have been recently, cover labour (for anaesthesia) with hydrocortisone (inhaled steroids do not need parenteral cover during labour).
- Status asthmaticus is treated by steroids in high doses, bronchodilators and artificial ventilation, if necessary.

PULMONARY TUBERCULOSIS

- If the diagnosis is made during pregnancy, treat with the standard regimen (pyrazinamide for 2 months and isoniazid with rifampicin for 6 months). Pyridoxine supplements are advised. Do not use streptomycin in pregnancy.
- Breast-feeding is contraindicated if the patient has sputum-positive TB.

- The infant requires BCG vaccination and should be separated from the mother only if she has open TB and until Mantoux conversion.

EPILEPSY

- Pre-pregnancy counselling is important for women with epilepsy in order to:
  —check their anticonvulsant therapy for need, safety and dosage
  —allay their many fears about pregnancy and nursing a small baby.
- Pregnancy does not provoke epilepsy in mothers but the frequency of seizures may increase because anticonvulsants are cleared more quickly.
- The risk of an epileptic mother having an epileptic baby is about 1/40.

TERATOGENICITY OF ANTICONVULSANTS

- The incidence of congenital malformations is increased two- to three-fold in infants of women on anticonvulsants.
- No one drug is free of risk, but phenytoin (alone or in combination) is implicated most frequently.
- Among the problems are:
  —cleft lip and/or palate (increased ten-fold)
  —congenital heart defect (increased four-fold)
  —hypoplasia of terminal phalanges of fingers
  —possible characteristic facial appearance: wide-spaced eyes, low posterior hair line, short neck, prominent brow and trigoncephaly
  —retarded growth, delayed development and, occasionally, mental retardation.
- Sodium valproate is associated with fetal spina bifida in about 1% of 'at risk' pregnancies.

MANAGEMENT

- Prescribe anticonvulsants in doses sufficient to prevent convulsions.
- Single-drug therapy should be aimed for if possible.
- Vitamin K should be given to all neonates (1 mg i.m.).
- Breast-feeding is not contraindicated.
- Status epilepticus is best treated with intravenous diazepam. The airway must be kept patent and oxygen administered.

DISEASES OF LIVER AND ALIMENTARY TRACT

JAUNDICE

Incidence approximately 1/1500 pregnancies.

JAUNDICE CAUSED BY PREGNANCY

Intrahepatic cholestasis (20% of cases)
- The patient has pruritus in the second half of pregnancy (some never become jaundiced).
- Bilirubin and transaminases are slightly elevated.
- It is associated with some increased risk of pre-term labour, fetal distress and perinatal death.
- It clears up after delivery and does not proceed to chronic liver disease.
- It tends to recur in subsequent pregnancies and may also occur in association with oestrogen-containing oral contraceptives.
- Cholestyramine will reduce itching but is very unpleasant to take. Parenteral vitamin K is required if jaundice causes prolongation of the prothrombin time.

Jaundice complicating pre-eclampsia—see page 67.

INTERCURRENT JAUNDICE IN PREGNANCY

Viral hepatitis (40% of cases)
Due either to hepatitis B or C (long incubation, serum hepatitis) or hepatitis A (short incubation, infective hepatitis). Hepatitis B is discussed on page 109.

Cholelithiasis (6% of cases)
- Modern ultrasound or transhepatic cholangiography may be useful in confirming the diagnosis.
- Cholecystectomy can be carried out in pregnancy if necessary, preferably not earlier or later than the second trimester.

Drug toxicity and haemolysis
These are rare causes, but should be considered.

PRE-EXISTING LIVER DISEASE

- Pregnancy is uncommon in the presence of cirrhosis due, for example, to active chronic hepatitis, or primary biliary cirrhosis.
- The prognosis is good for mother and baby in familial non-haemolytic jaundice, e.g. Gilbert's and the Dubin–Johnson syndromes. Pregnancy may increase jaundice in the latter.

GASTRIC REFLUX AND HIATUS HERNIA

The lower oesophageal sphincter relaxes under the influence of pregnancy hormones. Reflux of acid gastric contents leads to *heartburn*. This can also be due to a 'sliding' hiatus hernia.

Management
- Frequent small meals; advise patient to avoid lying flat; simple antacids.

- If no relief is obtained, 'floating' antacids, or metoclopramide, can be tried.

COELIAC DISEASE

- Coeliac disease may present in pregnancy as a folate deficiency anaemia.
- If untreated it may be associated with an increased risk of abortion or IUGR.
- It is successfully treated by a gluten-free diet and vitamin supplements.

ULCERATIVE COLITIS

- Ulcerative colitis does not affect pregnancy adversely.
- Pregnancy does not increase the chance of relapse of quiescent colitis, but if the colitis arises de novo in pregnancy or the puerperium it carries a poor prognosis.
- Treatment can continue during pregnancy with rectal and systemic steroids and/or sulphasalazine.
- In the presence of an ileostomy most pregnancies proceed to normal vaginal delivery.

CROHN'S DISEASE

- There may be a small adverse effect on fetal outcome due to the disease.
- The condition itself is usually unaffected by pregnancy.
- Deterioration is most likely in the puerperium.
- It should be managed in the same manner as in the non-pregnant.

PSYCHIATRIC DISORDERS

POSTPARTUM 'BLUES'

- This is not an illness but rather a transient mild disturbance characterised by:
  —weeping   —feelings of helplessness
  —irritability   —sensitivity to criticism
  —variation in mood   —poor sleep.
- It occurs in at least 50% of postpartum women, usually develops around the third day, and may last for a few hours or days.
- Treatment is by psychological support and reassurance.

DEPRESSIVE ILLNESS

- This is characterised by tiredness, lethargy, irritability and anxiety, which may be more prominent than depression.

- It is often brought on by psycho-social stress, and there may be a previous psychiatric history.
- Its peak incidence is 3 months postpartum.
- Treatment is by psychological and practical support and anti-depressant drugs as necessary.

PUERPERAL PSYCHOSIS

- The incidence is about 2/1000 livebirths.
- Puerperal psychosis presents either as an affective disorder with depression or hypomania, or schizophrenia with delusions and hallucinations.
- It often begins within 4 days of delivery.
- A psychiatrist must be consulted because there is risk of suicide and harm to or neglect of the baby.
- There is an increased risk of psychotic illness in the future, including during further pregnancies.
- Monoamine oxidase inhibitors are best avoided in pregnancy, but withdrawal must be gradual.

THROMBOSIS AND THROMBOEMBOLISM

COAGULATION AND FIBRINOLYSIS DURING NORMAL PREGNANCY (see p. 99)

- Factors VII, VIII, IX and X are increased from the beginning of the second trimester. The most marked increase is in plasma fibrinogen. This results in a relative hypercoagulable state ready to cope with placental separation at delivery.
- Plasma fibrinolytic activity is decreased because plasmin inhibitors (e.g. α_2-macroglobulin and α_1-antitrypsin) increase substantially.
- Fibrinolysis returns to normal within 15 minutes of delivery of the placenta.

MATERNAL MORTALITY FROM THROMBOSIS AND THROMBOEMBOLISM (TE)

- These were the commonest causes of maternal death in the UK from 1991–93, making up over 25% of the total.
- Of the 35 deaths, 30 were from *pulmonary thromboembolism* (PTE) and five from *cerebral thrombosis*. Another five deaths from PTE occurred beyond the 42nd day.
- In the deaths from PTE, 12 occurred antepartum, one intrapartum and 17 postpartum.
- Of the 17 postpartum PTE deaths, 13 (76%) followed caesarean section, as did all five from cerebral thrombosis.

FACTORS ASSOCIATED WITH INCREASED RISK

- **Slight increase in risk**—requires early mobilisation and hydration:
  —elective caesarean section in an uncomplicated pregnancy with no other risk markers
  —blood groups other than O.
- **Moderate increase in risk**—consider prophylaxis (see below):
  —maternal age >35 years. The risk in women aged over 40 years is 60 times that for those aged 25 or less
  —parity 4 or more
  —obesity (>80 kg) associated with poor mobility and venous stasis
  —gross varicose veins
  —proteinuric pre-eclampsia
  —any surgical procedure in labour (particularly emergency caesarean section)
  —immobility before surgery (>4 days)
  —sickle cell disease, major intercurrent illness or infection.
- **High risk**—requires heparin and leg stockings (see below):
  —three or more moderate risk factors
  —personal or family history of thrombosis. The risk of recurrence in a woman with a past history of thromboembolism occurring in pregnancy or while on 'the pill' is about 12%, the majority of which are postnatal
  —'thrombophilia', i.e. antithrombin III, protein C or protein S deficiencies; activated protein C resistance (due to the presence of factor V Leiden)
  —anti-cardiolipin syndrome or presence of lupus inhibitor
  —major surgery, e.g. caesarean hysterectomy.

INCIDENCE

- The incidence of non-fatal TE in pregnancy is not known.
- *Deep vein thrombosis (DVT)* complicates about 2% of caesarean sections.

Deep vein thrombosis

- The most common clinical features are pain, local tenderness, swelling, oedema, a positive Homan's sign, a change in leg colour and temperature and a palpable thrombosed vein.
- Most cases are less obvious and some are silent. Clinical diagnosis is therefore unreliable.
- Over 80% are left-sided.
- (*Superficial thrombophlebitis* does not carry a significant risk of thromboembolism unless it extends to the deep veins.)

DIAGNOSIS

- Venography is the 'gold standard'.
- Ultrasonic detection of venous patency is inadequate.

- Radioactive fibrinogen uptake is contraindicated.

The main complications are pulmonary embolism and chronic vascular insufficiency.

Pulmonary embolism
There may be no prior clinical evidence of DVT.

Signs and symptoms. Pleuritic pain, haemoptysis, dyspnoea and varying degrees of shock. Consider also if there is no other obvious explanation for tachycardia, pyrexia or bronchospasm.

Investigation
- Chest X-ray may be helpful but can be totally normal.
- ECG—usually normal except when the embolus is large and has produced acute cor pulmonale. Even these changes may be obscured by the usual ECG changes which occur in pregnancy.
- Ventilation-perfusion isotope (VQ) lung scan.
- Pulmonary angiography may need to be considered.

MANAGEMENT OF DVT AND PULMONARY EMBOLISM

Heparin does not cross the placenta or reach breast milk so there is no added risk to the fetus. Its action is to inhibit thrombin and factors IX, X, XI and XII.
- Acute therapy—intravenous calcium heparin 40 000 units daily (in saline by infusion pump) for at least 48 hours.
- Long-term therapy—subcutaneous heparin inhibits activated factor X without prolonging the clotting time. Use a twice-daily unfractionated heparin *or* a single daily dose of low molecular weight heparin. This does not add to the risk of haemorrhage even at caesarean section. Continue for at least 6 weeks postpartum (or warfarin may be substituted after delivery).
- Side-effects of long-term therapy include allergic reactions, thrombocytopenia and maternal osteopenia, which is dose- and duration-dependent with some unpredictable individual susceptibility.

Warfarin inhibits the synthesis of vitamin K-dependent clotting factors (II, VII, IX and X). It crosses the placenta readily but not significantly in breast milk.
- It is best avoided in the first trimester because of a slight risk of embryopathy.
- Even with meticulous control (prothrombin time 2–2.5 times the clotting time for a normal control plasma), there is an increased risk of fetal haemorrhage.
- Its anticoagulant effect cannot be reversed rapidly.
- Therefore heparin therapy is preferred unless the benefits of warfarin outweigh the risks.

- Because of the increased risk of haemorrhage if warfarin is used, change to heparin at 36 weeks' gestation. If labour supervenes while the patient is taking warfarin it can be counteracted with fresh frozen plasma.
- Breast-feeding is not contraindicated.
- Warfarin should be continued for at least 6 weeks after delivery.

Dextran 70 The risks of anaphylaxis to the mother and subsequent uterine hypertonus to the fetus may exceed any benefit. Therefore its use is best avoided during pregnancy.

Aspirin and other anti-platelet agents Prophylactic efficacy has not been assessed.

PROPHYLAXIS OF THROMBOEMBOLISM

The following is a guide to policy.
- **Women at high risk of TE** (see above): use long-term subcutaneous heparin (unfractionated 7500–10 000 units 12-hourly *or* low mol. weight 40 mg/day); also consider graduated elastic compression stockings. Commence 4–6 weeks before gestation at which any previous TE occurred and continue for at least 6 weeks postpartum.
- **Women with thrombophilia**
  —Obtain expert haematological advice
  —For protein S or C deficiency or anti-cardiolipin syndrome, use above regime
  —For antithrombin III deficiency the level of risk is such that the heparin dose should be controlled by anti-factor Xa measurements (target levels 0.2–0.4 i.u./ml) in discussion with haematology. Antithrombin III can be given to cover the further risk at delivery.
- **Previous episode in pregnancy** without other risk markers— consider antenatal prophylaxis and give subcutaneous heparin (unfractionated 5000 units 12-hourly or low mol. weight 20 mg daily) or warfarin for at least 6 weeks postpartum.
- **Women at moderate risk**—management depends on extent of perceived risk. In general, treat postnatally but also consider antenatally if single risk is marked or more than one is present (e.g. treat women with history of TE who are admitted to hospital for bed rest).
- **Regional anaesthesia?**—epidural or spinal block is contraindicated if patient is fully anticoagulated. However, there is no evidence that prophylactic heparin increases the risk of spinal haematoma. Each case must be judged on its merits but the following guidelines are suggested:
  —delay siting of block for 4–6 h after last dose of heparin?
  —*or* delay heparin until block is sited?

—*or* delay heparin until after the delivery or operation?

For further discussion see Further Reading.

MALIGNANT DISEASE AND PREGNANCY

Pregnancy does not usually adversely affect the course of malignant disease. The poor prognosis of pregnant women with cervical cancer is more likely to be due to the aggressiveness of the tumour in women in that age group than to the pregnancy itself.

CERVICAL CANCER AND CERVICAL INTRAEPITHELIAL NEOPLASIA

- Offer a cervical smear at the booking antenatal clinic if the women has never had one before or not within the past 5 years.
- If the smear is abnormal carry out colposcopy (colposcopically-directed biopsies can be taken safely in pregnancy).

Cervical intraepithelial neoplasia (CIN) should be serially observed for the remainder of pregnancy and dealt with definitively at the end of the puerperium.

Invasive carcinoma of the cervix

The condition poses several clinical problems in pregnancy.
- If discovered under 22 weeks' gestation advise termination (by hysterotomy) followed by definitive treatment (see p. 270).
- Between 22 and 26 weeks it may be justifiable to await fetal viability before ending the pregnancy.
- Thereafter, delivery should be effected in consultation with a neonatal paediatrician and the woman herself.
- Vaginal delivery is contraindicated.

Whatever the management, the prognosis is poor.

OVARIAN CANCER

- Ovarian tumours of all varieties are said to complicate 1/1000 pregnancies, although only 1 in 20 are malignant. The frequency of tumour types is as in the non-pregnant woman (see p. 285).
- Ultrasound is useful for detection of ovarian swellings.

Management

- Treat as in the non-pregnant woman (see p. 291).
- The prognosis seems to be better for ovarian cancer in pregnancy, with a 5-year survival rate of up to 75% compared to an overall 25%. This reflects the nature of the tumours in this age group.

BREAST CANCER

- This is the commonest malignant tumour to affect women. About 2% of women under 45 years of age who have the disease are pregnant at the time of diagnosis.
- Lymph node involvement seems to be increased in pregnancy. Prognosis may therefore be poorer.

Management

- In the first half of pregnancy, treatment should be as for the non-pregnant woman; if chemotherapy is necessary, termination is advisable.
- In the second half of pregnancy, delivery should be effected if the fetus is viable; treatment can then begin. It may be justifiable to delay treatment for a short time to await fetal viability in some cases.
- Breast-feeding is probably contraindicated.
- Further pregnancies can be embarked on if desired after a post-treatment interval of at least 2 years.

HODGKIN'S DISEASE

This affects about 1 in 6000 pregnant women.

Management

- In the first half of pregnancy radiotherapy can be carried out with shielding of the uterus and ovaries.
- In later pregnancy chemo- and radiotherapy can sometimes be delayed until after delivery.

MELANOMA

- Pregnancy appears to have no significant influence on survival.
- Pregnancy is probably best avoided for 3 years following excision because most recurrences arise within that time.
- Management of a melanoma found in pregnancy is as for the non-pregnant woman.
- Transplacental spread to the fetus can occur but is exceedingly rare.

FURTHER READING

Creasy R K, Resnik R (eds) 1994 Maternal–fetal medicine—principles and practice. Saunders, Philadelphia

Greer I A 1989 Thromboembolic problems in pregnancy. Fetal Medicine Review 1:79–103

Oats J N (ed) 1991 Diabetes in pregnancy. Clinical Obstetrics and Gynaecology. Baillière Tindall, London

RCOG Working Party on Prophylaxis against Thromboembolism in Gynaecology and Obstetrics 1995: Report. RCOG, London

Scott J R, Stirrat G M 1992 The immune system in disease. Clinical Obstetrics and Gynaecology 6:393–679

Tan E M et al 1982 The 1982 revised criteria for the classification of systemic lupus erythematosus. Arthritis and Rheumatism 25:1271–1277

THRIFT Consensus Group 1992 Risk of and prophylaxis for venous thromboembolism in hospital patients. British Medical Journal 305:567–574

8. Maternal and fetal infections

NON-SEXUALLY TRANSMITTED VIRAL INFECTIONS
RUBELLA

Naturally acquired infection confers life-long immunity.

Prevention by vaccination
- The policy of routine vaccination of girls in their early teens has made a major contribution to prevention of rubella infection in pregnancy.
- Antenatal testing for rubella antibody should be routine even when noted to be positive in a previous pregnancy.
- Non-immune women should be offered vaccination within 7 days of delivery.
- The vaccine is a live-attenuated virus and, although no cases of fetal rubella infection have been noted after vaccination, it should be avoided for 3 months before and during pregnancy.
- Accidental vaccination during pregnancy is not an indication for termination.

Clinical features
- The incubation period is 14–18 days. Affected women are infectious for the last week of incubation and the first week after the rash appears. Only laboratory tests can confirm that a rash is due to rubella.
- The virus damages mitosis, which retards cell division. Major malformations are likely if infection occurs during the critical stage of organogenesis.
- The frequency of congenital infection after maternal rubella with a rash is:
  —>80% in the first trimester
  —50% at 13–14 weeks
  —25% at the end of the second trimester.
- Among the congenital defects associated (singly or in combination) with maternal rubella are:
  —cardiac lesions of many kinds
  —eye lesions—cataract, chorioretinitis, microphthalmia, glaucoma
  —deafness
  —an 'expanded syndrome' involving the liver, spleen, brain and

skeleton which may lead to abortion, stillbirth, IUGR, microcephaly, or mental retardation.
- Rubella-associated defects are present in almost all infants infected before 11 weeks (mainly cardiac lesions and deafness), and in 35% of those infected at 13–16 weeks (mainly deafness). Infection after 16 weeks is not usually associated with defects.

Management after maternal exposure
- Test the mother for rubella-specific IgM.
- If there is no antibody or only low titres, repeat the tests 25–28 days after exposure.
  —No rise is reassuring
  —A rise in titre of four-fold or more confirms recent infection.
- If infection is confirmed, advice will depend on the gestation.
  —In early pregnancy chorionic villus sampling (CVS) (see p. 51) can be used to locate the rubella virus in the placenta/fetus by in situ hybridisation
  —In later pregnancy CVS can be considered. Monitor fetal growth and welfare.

CYTOMEGALOVIRUS (CMV)

- CMV is the commonest primary viral infection of pregnant women. It is usually subclinical (95%).
- It may account for up to 10% of mental retardation in children up to 6 years of age.

CMV: other consequences	
Generalised effects	Abortion, stillbirth, IUGR, failure to thrive
Neurological effects	Microcephaly, cerebral palsy, optic atrophy, deafness
Other effects	Thrombocytopenic purpura, jaundice, pneumonia

- The information box lists some other consequences of CMV.
- However, of congenitally infected infants, less than 10% have serious handicaps, and only a minority of these could be detected before 28 weeks.
- Congenital infection follows primary (75%) or reinfection (25%) of the mother.
- In light of this, and since no treatment is available, routine screening of pregnant women to detect evidence of primary infection is not clinically useful.
- The virus is excreted in breast milk.
- Only CMV-negative blood should be used for transfusion in sero-negative pregnant women and all newborn infants.

VARICELLA ZOSTER (CHICKENPOX)

- Over 80% of children have had chickenpox by 10 years of age and >85% of adults who cannot remember having it are immune on testing.
- The incidence of primary infections during pregnancy is 0.5–0.7/1000 pregnancies.
- The effects on the mother range from the typical rash to life-threatening viral pneumonitis (rarely).
- About 2% of fetuses are affected if maternal infection occurs in the first 20 weeks of pregnancy. The *congenital varicella syndrome* may include:
  —scarring (with dermatomal distribution)
  —eye defects
  —hypoplasia of bone and muscle of a limb (usually on same side as scarring)
  —neurological abnormalities (mental retardation, microcephaly, dysfunction of bowel and bladder sphincters).
- Zoster immune globulin should be given to affected women in early pregnancy and to the infants of women affected in late pregnancy.

HUMAN PARVOVIRUS B19

- This causes 'erythema infectiosum' (Fifth disease or 'slapped cheek syndrome') possibly preceded by a non-specific febrile illness.
- The incidence is <1% of pregnancies.
- Most women with B19 infection in pregnancy have a normal infant but it may inhibit fetal erythropoiesis. This can cause severe fetal anaemia, ascites and hydrops which can be corrected by intrauterine transfusion.

SEXUALLY TRANSMITTED DISEASES (STDs)

Human papillomavirus (HPV—wart virus)
- This is the commonest STD.
- Warts tend to grow in pregnancy—they can be treated by trichloracetic acid.

HERPES SIMPLEX VIRUS (HSV)

- HSV Type 2 causes 70% of herpetic genital-tract infections. Small vulval or vaginal vesicles may become painful ulcers. Diagnosis is by culture in special viral culture medium. Acyclovir cream reduces the duration of signs and symptoms.
- The fetus has no intrinsic immunity to the virus and no passive immunity during a primary maternal infection. Transmission of herpes infection from mother to the fetus/baby is high (40%)

after vaginal delivery in primary maternal infection, but low (3%) if infection is recurrent.
- The following policy is therefore suggested.

Primary infection with active genital lesions:
—delivery by caesarean section if labour occurs and if membranes intact, or within 4 hours of membrane rupture. Take viral swabs from baby (treat with acyclovir if positive)
—if more than 4 hours since membrane rupture allow vaginal delivery because caesarean section will not reduce risk of neonatal infection. Take viral swabs from baby and treat him/her with acyclovir.

Secondary infection with active genital lesions:
—although the perceived risk of neonatal infection is much less, its extent is not fully known. The above policy tends to be adopted in the absence of good evidence to the contrary.
- Asymptomatic viral shedding is neither predictable nor preventable. A diagnosis of neonatal herpes should be considered if the infant becomes ill unexpectedly in the first weeks of life even in the absence of risk factors for HSV infection.

HEPATITIS B VIRUS (HBV)

- Most adults recover fully and become immune after HBV infection. 10% become carriers.
- All pregnant women should be routinely screened for the HBV surface antigen (HBsAg) at booking (or when they present if previously unscreened).
- The fetus is at risk if the mother:
  —has recently had acute HBV infection (which may have been asymptomatic)
  —carries the surface antigen (HBsAg+), is positive for the core antigen (eAg+) but has not developed antibodies to it (eAb–) *or* is eAg–/eAb–.
- Carriers who have antibodies to the e antigen of the virus (eAb+) are not infectious but should not be blood donors.
- Risks of transmission to fetus are given in the box.

Maternal immune status	Risk of transmission to fetus
eAg+	90%
eAg–/eAb–	40%
eAb+	10%

- Infants of HBsAG-positive mothers should be given Hep.B gammaglobulin (HBIG) within 12 hours of birth and an initial

dose of HBV vaccine within 7 days. Give further doses of vaccine at 1 and 6 months. Test for HBsAg at 12–15 months.
- Advice about breast-feeding is controversial.

HEPATITIS C VIRUS (HCV)

- This is the major cause of non-A, non-B post-transfusion hepatitis and a frequent cause of sporadic hepatitis in the USA and Western Europe.
- The risk of sexual transmission is much lower than for HBV but the inoculation risk (IR) categories are as shown below (p. 000).
- Up to 80% of those infected become chronic carriers, with many progressing slowly to chronic active hepatitis and cirrhosis.
- The acute phase is often asymptomatic.
- Vertical transmission during pregnancy is much less likely than with HBV (with the possible exception of HIV+ women).
- Routine screening for HCV in pregnancy is currently unwarranted.
- Pregnant women at high risk of HCV infection should have antibody testing and their infants should be observed for the development of hepatitis.
- HCV infection does not seem to increase the risk of pregnancy complications, nor does pregnancy have any effect on HCV hepatitis.
- Although severe HCV infections have been successfully treated with α-interferon, this should not be used in pregnancy because of the risk of maternal side-effects and unknown effects on the fetus.

HUMAN IMMUNODEFICIENCY VIRUS (HIV) INFECTION

See Further Reading for fuller discussion.
- HIV infections are most commonly acquired in Europe through i.v. drug abuse. Heterosexually acquired AIDS is not common in the UK but is increasing among women with a partner in a 'high risk' group (see below).
- In some areas in sub-Saharan Africa 10–30% of pregnant women are HIV infected and the incidence is increasing rapidly in SE Asia.
- The risk of mother to child transmission ranges from about 15 to 30% with lowest rates in Europe and highest in Africa.
- Transmission depends on many factors, e.g. viral load and biological/genetic variation of HIV; presence of neutralising antibody; presence of chorio-amnionitis or other STDs; mode of delivery; and breast-feeding.
- Pregnancy may increase the progression to symptomatic infection by accelerating the depletion of helper T lymphocytes and the resulting immunodeficiency.

Antenatal HIV testing

- Voluntary testing (with counselling) particularly of 'high-risk' women (see below) provides the opportunity to reduce risk of transmission and offer prophylactic treatment. The adverse consequences (e.g. anxiety, stigma and possible discrimination) need to be considered. *It must, therefore, be with informed consent*.
- About 50% of women found to be HIV infected during pregnancy are likely to progress to AIDS or the AIDS Related Complex (ARC) in 2–6 years.
- Special precautions should still be taken in handling blood and other body fluids from women at 'high risk' who refuse HIV testing (see below).

Vertical transmission

- HIV infection can occur in utero, during labour or delivery and from breast-feeding:
  —intrauterine infection is defined by detection of HIV in blood from the infant (by culture or polymerase chain reaction) within 48 hours of birth
  —intrapartum infection is presumed when test results are negative in the first week of life but become positive between days 7 and 90 in an infant who is not breast-fed
  —these definitions need to be kept under review
  —probably about 70% of transmission occurs in late pregnancy and labour.

Reduction of vertical transmission

- Treatment of other STDs
- Anti-retroviral therapy (e.g. zidovudine) for the mother during pregnancy/delivery and for the infant after birth
- Reduction in peripartum exposure, e.g:
  —delivery by caesarean section for HIV-positive women? The European Collaborative Study (see Further Reading) suggested a 50% reduction in transmission with this policy. This is currently being studied further
  —avoidance of intrapartum invasive procedures, e.g. fetal scalp electrode or blood sampling
- Avoidance of breast-feeding wherever possible—in developing countries the risk of *not* breast-feeding may be the greater
- Passive immunotherapy for baby and/or mother is being evaluated. Active immunisation is undergoing preliminary studies in the USA.

INOCULATION RISK (IR) WOMEN

- The information box gives those women with an increased likelihood of carrying hepatitis B virus, HIV or other agents spread by inoculation.

Inoculation risk women	
• Known or suspected AIDS or ARC	• Childhood spent in developing world[2]
• HIV antibody-positive	• Visit to Central Africa in past 5 years[2]
• HBsAg-positive/anti HBe-negative	• Treated using blood products[2]
• History of acute hepatitis in past 6 weeks[1]	• Sexual partners of HIV risk men[2]
	• Intravenous drug abusers
• Chronic active hepatitis or cirrhosis[1]	

[1]Can be excluded if found to be HBsAg-negative but eAg+ and eAb+
[2]Can be excluded if HIV-negative and more than 1 year since last exposure

- Babies of HIV-positive mothers are also at risk.
- All blood or other body fluids being sent to laboratories from IR women must be clearly identified. All personnel dealing with IR women should be immunised against HBV.

RISK TO MEDICAL AND NURSING PERSONNEL

- The risk of HIV seroconversion after a single needlestick or sharps injury is <0.5%.
- Without vaccination, the risk of acquiring hepatitis B from an HBeAg+ patient after a single exposure by needlestick or sharps injury may be as high as 30%.
- *All personnel at risk must be vaccinated against HBV* (and seroconversion confirmed).

CARE OF IR WOMEN IN LABOUR AND POSTNATALLY

- Make sure there is a well defined policy for caring for all IR patients including those HIV positive.
- It is advised that those looking after IR women in labour should:
  —wear adequate eye protection, protective clothing and double gloves, particularly for operative delivery
  —avoid needlestick injuries
  —handle body fluids with care and dispose of soiled garments as per above policy
  —sterilise instruments by autoclave.
- Try to avoid use of fetal scalp clip and sampling to minimise risk of transmission to neonate.
- Warn paediatricians of forthcoming delivery.
- Avoid mouth-operated suction devices.

TREPONEMAL INFECTIONS

- Syphilis, yaws and pinta are all caused by treponemes which are indistinguishable morphologically and serologically.

- Clinically apparent syphilis is rare in pregnancy in the UK but failure to diagnose it can have severe long-term effects on mother and child. Routine antenatal screening is therefore still indicated and cost-effective.
- Syphilis is still rife in developing countries.

Screening for syphilis
- Blood is taken at booking for VDRL (Venereal Disease Reference Laboratory) or RPR (Reiter protein reagin) and TPHA (*Treponema pallidum* haemagglutination) test.
- More specific testing is necessary if screening tests are positive, there is a history of contact or there is clinical evidence of syphilis.
- FTA[abs] (fluorescent treponemal antibody-absorbed) test is the most sensitive for syphilis.

Biological false-positive reactions (BFPR) are much commoner than true infections and may occur spontaneously in pregnancy, after blood transfusion or recent vaccination as well as many other conditions (e.g. SLE). FTA[abs] is negative in BFPR detected by other tests.

Treatment of syphilis
- Use penicillin unless the patient is allergic. (If allergy is mild use cephaloridine: if severe, use erythromycin.)
- It may be best to re-treat women in subsequent pregnancies.

Congenital syphilis
- Syphilis can have serious effects on every organ and system in the developing fetus and early maternal syphilis carries a high rate of fetal infection.
- Adequate treatment of the mother before 16 weeks of pregnancy will prevent infection in virtually all cases. Treatment after this time will still be effective in most cases.

OTHER INFECTIONS
GROUP B STREPTOCOCCAL (GBS) INFECTION

- In the UK, 15–20% of women carry GBS in the vagina at delivery.
- 40–70% of infants of mothers colonised antenatally with GBS are themselves colonised, but only 1% develop evidence of infection affected by it.
- Nevertheless GBS infections are one of the commonest infective causes of neonatal morbidity and mortality in the developed world with an incidence of 1–4/1000 births.
- Among the particular risk factors for the fetus are:
  —premature rupture of membranes before 37 weeks
  —rupture of membranes for >18 hours at any gestational age

—multiple births
—maternal pyrexia in labour
—a previous affected child.
- The mortality rate for perinatal infection can be as high as 80% despite early recognition and prompt treatment.
- Routine screening for maternal colonisation and treatment if GBS-positive is controversial. The American Association of Pediatrics (AAP) has recommended routine screening at 26–28 weeks with intrapartum antibiotic therapy for colonised women who have any of the above risk factors. However, review of the evidence so far (see Further Reading) suggests that:
  —GBS is only temporarily eradicated by short-term antibiotic therapy during pregnancy
  —if treatment is based on a positive culture at 28 weeks up to 50% will be negative at delivery; and up to 15% of culture-negative women at 28 weeks will be culture-positive by delivery. Thus some women would be overtreated while others would be undertreated.
- The current conclusion, which must be kept under review, is that *there is insufficient firm evidence to support routine screening for GBS during pregnancy and antibiotic treatment for women found to be positive.*
- However, the presence of GBS in the vagina after premature rupture of the membranes may be an indication for delivery and treatment of the infant.

GROUP A STREPTOCOCCAL (GAS) INFECTION

- GAS septicaemia caused five maternal deaths in the UK from 1991–93. All patients died of respiratory or multi-organ failure within 24 hours of becoming ill.
- These cases illustrate the virulence of GAS even in the modern antibiotic era.

BACTERIAL VAGINOSIS (BV)

- This is due to replacement of the normal vaginal flora predominantly with anaerobes, as is described on page 261.
- Its presence has been associated with a ×2 increase in intra-amniotic infection and pre-term birth.
- Treatment for *symptomatic* BV during pregnancy can be with intravaginal clindamycin cream or metronidazole gel.
- The effect of treatment on *asymptomatic* women with BV has not yet been fully evaluated.

TOXOPLASMOSIS

- Toxoplasmosis is a systemic infection caused by the protozoon *Toxoplasma gondii*. It is either asymptomatic or confused with 'flu' or other pregnancy symptoms.

- The best estimate of the incidence in pregnant women in the UK is about 2/1000.
- When acquired in pregnancy it can cause fetal infection with potentially severe sequelae such as cerebral calcification, hydrocephalus and chorioretinitis. The risks vary according to gestational age at infection:
  —during the first trimester transmission to the fetus occurs in about 10% of infections. Fetal death or severe sequelae are likely
  —during the second trimester transmission is frequent with a high risk of congenital infection
  —during the third trimester transmission is very frequent but the risk of problems at birth is low. However, as many as 80% of children may develop chorioretinitis in later years.
- The best policy is prevention by avoiding undercooked meat, unpasteurised milk, and contact with cat litter; washing all garden produce well and washing hands after gardening.

TESTING AND TREATING THE MOTHER

- Routine screening is not of proven benefit in the UK in light of current knowledge (see Further Reading). This needs to be kept under review.
- Serological testing should be carried out on suspicion, looking for specific IgM antibody. If positive, repeat for confirmation and to check for rising antibody titres.
- If current infection is confirmed, treatment of the mother with spiramycin for the remainder of pregnancy will reduce transplacental infection by 60%.

TESTING AND TREATING THE FETUS

- If current infection is confirmed in the mother, consider the following:
  —carry out amniocentesis and cordocentesis. Infection is confirmed if these samples contain specific IgM antibodies
  —check for ventricular dilatation by ultrasound at 20–22 weeks
  —if the fetus is infected and ventricular dilatation is present counsel couple regarding termination
  —if fetus is infected but seems normal, or parents do not wish to consider termination, treat with pyrimethamine, sulphadiazine and folinic acid for 3 weeks alternating with spiramycin for 3 weeks for remainder of pregnancy
  —continue ultrasound monitoring of ventricles.
- After birth:
  —send samples of placenta, amniotic fluid, cord and maternal blood for serology
  —carry out detailed clinical examination including cranial X-ray and ultrasound and ophthalmoscopy

—if toxoplasmosis suspected, treat as above for 1 year.
- A further pregnancy can be embarked on once the anti-Toxoplasma IgM has disappeared. This can take from 6 months to 2 years.

LISTERIOSIS

- Caused by *Listeria monocytogenes*, which is widely distributed
- Rate of listeriosis is about 1 in 10 000 births in the UK
- Source is usually dairy products, vegetables, meat and meat products (e.g. paté), poultry or shellfish. Pasteurisation may not eradicate the organism. It thrives at 4°C (see Further Reading)
- Should be considered in all cases of 'flu'-like pyrexial illness in pregnancy, mid-trimester miscarriage or pre-term delivery (particularly if amniotic fluid is meconium-stained)
- If suspected, take vaginal swabs for Gram staining and culture, and blood cultures
- After birth, placenta should be examined for the organism
- A live-born infant may develop a generalised infection, including meningitis and pneumonia
- Organism is sensitive to a wide range of antibiotics including ampicillin.

TUBERCULOSIS

- Among those for whom screening for TB infection should be considered in pregnancy are:
  —women in close contact with a known or suspected case
  —those recently arrived from an endemic area, e.g. Africa or Asia
  —women who are HIV + and/or i.v. drug abusers.
- Diagnosis is confirmed by PPD skin testing, chest X-ray and three sputum samples.

Treatment
- Active disease—use isoniazid (INH) with rifampicin, or ethambutol (or both) and continue until course is completed.
- If PPD+ but no other evidence of active disease, consider INH prophylaxis.
- If INH is prescribed, monitor liver function and give pyridoxine supplements to reduce risk of CNS toxicity.
- The baby should receive BCG vaccination. Breast-feeding is *not* contraindicated.

MALARIA

- Malaria must be considered in non-endemic areas among immigrants or tourists returning from endemic areas suffering from unexplained pyrexia.

- Parasites are seen on thick and thin blood smears.
- Treat with chloroquine if possible.
- Advise pregnant women to avoid travel to endemic areas, especially those with drug-resistant strains. If such travel is unavoidable, prophylaxis is strongly advised.

FURTHER READING

Burrow G N, Ferris T F 1995 Medical complications during pregnancy, 4th edn. Saunders, Philadelphia

The Cochrane Collaboration 1995 Cochrane Pregnancy & Childbirth Database, Issue 2. BMJ Publications, London

Connor E M et al 1994 Reduction of maternal–infant transmission of HIV-1 with Zidovudine treatment. New England Journal of Medicine 331:1173–1180

Creasy R K, Resnik R (eds) 1994 Maternal–fetal medicine—principles and practice, 3rd edn. Saunders, Philadelphia

European Collaborative Study on Risk Factors for Mother to Child Transmission of HIV-1 1992 Report. Lancet 339:1007–1012

Hibbard B M, Anderson M A, Drife J O, Tighe J R et al 1996 Report on confidential enquiries into maternal deaths in the United Kingdom 1991–93. HMSO, London

James D K, Steer P J, Weiner C P, Gonik B (eds) 1994 High risk pregnancy—management options. Saunders, London

Johnstone F D (ed) 1992 HIV infection in obstetrics and gynaecology. Clinical Obstetrics and Gynaecology 6:1–216

Ohlsson A, Myhr T L 1994 Intrapartum prophylaxis of perinatal GBS infections: a critical review of RCTs. American Journal of Obstetrics and Gynaecology 170:910–917

Peckham C, Gibb D 1995 Mother to child transmission of HIV. New England Journal of Medicine 333:298–302

RCOG 1992 Prenatal screening for toxoplasmosis in the UK. Report of a Multidisciplinary Working Party. RCOG, London

Standing Medical Advisory Committee 1992 The diagnosis and treatment of suspected listeriosis in pregnancy—Report of a Working Group. Standing Medical Advisory Committee, London

Towers C V 1995 GBS: the US controversy. Lancet 346:197–199

9. Other pregnancy problems

ANTEPARTUM HAEMORRHAGE (APH)

Definition
Bleeding from the genital tract from 24 completed weeks of pregnancy to the birth of the baby, including the first and second stages of labour.

SOURCES

- Separation of a placenta lying partly or wholly within the lower uterine segment—*placenta praevia*
- Separation of a normally situated placenta—*abruptio placentae*
- Lesions of the cervix or vagina
- Unknown.

INCIDENCE

2–5% of pregnancies progressing beyond 24 weeks' gestation.

PLACENTA PRAEVIA

Definition
The placenta lies partially or wholly within the lower uterine segment. The simplest clinical classification is *minor degree* (placenta encroaches on lower segment but does not cover internal os) and *major degree* (placenta covers internal os).

MATERNAL RISKS

Among them are:
- *postpartum haemorrhage*—the risk is increased because of the less efficient contractility of the lower uterine segment
- *abnormally adherent placenta* (*placenta accreta*—see p. 164)—may occur in about 15% of women with placenta praevia. If the woman has been delivered by caesarean section in a previous pregnancy there is a risk of *placenta percreta*, in which the trophoblast has invaded through the entire thickness of the myometrium
- *anaesthetic and surgical complications*—more likely if caesarean section is carried out by inexperienced medical personnel as an emergency in face of major haemorrhage

- *recurrence*—4–8% of women who have had placenta praevia in one pregnancy will have it again in the next
- *maternal death*—there were four direct deaths due to placenta praevia in the UK between 1991 and 1993.

FETAL RISKS

Among them are:
- *prematurity*
- *IUGR*, particularly if multiple episodes of bleeding
- *fetal haemorrhage*—may be life-threatening if a fetal placental vessel crosses the cervical os and ruptures (*vasa praevia*): see Apt's test below
- both placenta praevia and abruption are associated with a two-fold increase in risk of *congenital malformations*.

CLINICAL FEATURES

- Vaginal bleeding—slight, moderate or heavy, most commonly occurring between 32 and 37 weeks' gestation.
- The bleeding is usually painless (in the absence of labour).
- It may have been preceded by several slight 'warning haemorrhages'.
- The abdomen is usually soft and non-tender to palpation, and the fetal heart can be heard.
- The presenting part is high, or the lie is oblique or transverse; breech presentation is common. (A persistently high presenting part or variable lie should raise the suspicion of *placenta praevia* even in the absence of vaginal bleeding.)

Management

- From home: organise immediate admission. *Do not perform a vaginal examination* because it may provoke profuse bleeding. Stop oral intake—mother may need an anaesthetic.
- In hospital: manage expectantly if haemorrhage is not severe and pregnancy has not reached 36–37 weeks:
  —localise placenta by ultrasound (see below)
  —a gentle speculum examination can be carried out when bleeding has ceased for at least 24 hours
  —keep 2 units of blood cross-matched as clinical judgment dictates
  —if bleeding continues make sure that the blood is maternal rather than fetal, using Apt's test, which distinguishes between them on the basis that fetal haemoglobin is relatively resistant to denaturation
  —check for feto-maternal transfusion in Rh-D-negative women and give anti-D immunoglobulin as necessary
  —monitor fetal welfare (see p. 57)

—if the diagnosis of significant placenta praevia is confirmed, the patient should remain in hospital.

INDICATIONS FOR INTERVENTION

- Heavy bleeding or continuous oozing is compromising maternal or fetal health.
- Moderate or heavy bleeding occurs when the pregnancy has reached 37 completed weeks or more.
- Expectant management has allowed the pregnancy to reach 38 weeks.

MODE OF INTERVENTION

- If the diagnosis of a major degree of placenta praevia is certain and maternal and/or fetal health are in jeopardy, or if there is a malpresentation, carry out caesarean section.
- If there is some doubt as to the diagnosis or the degree of placenta praevia is minor and the fetus presents by the vertex, carry out an examination in the theatre set for caesarean section.
- If placenta praevia is confirmed, proceed to caesarean section
- If not, an amniotomy can be performed.

LOCALISATION OF THE PLACENTA

- Ultrasound is the method of choice.
- If a low-lying placenta is detected early in pregnancy the scans should be repeated later in pregnancy (about 32 weeks?) because the placenta may seem to 'migrate' away from the lower segment as it forms in late pregnancy. Only 1 in 10 placentae thought to be low-lying early in pregnancy persists as clinically relevant placenta praevia towards term.
- A low-lying placenta discovered during an ultrasound examination for another reason and in the absence of bleeding can be managed as follows:
  —before 28 weeks—repeat the scan in 1 month
  —after 28 weeks—discuss the findings with the patient and advise her to avoid coitus. If she lives a long distance from the hospital, or if there are other adverse circumstances, it may be advisable to admit her to hospital. Repeat the scan each month.

ABRUPTIO PLACENTAE

Definition

- Haemorrhage arising from a normally situated placenta.
- *Revealed haemorrhage*—the blood tracks between the membrane and the uterine wall and escapes at the introitus.
- *Concealed haemorrhage*—a large haematoma forms between the placenta and the uterus. No external bleeding occurs.

- *Mixed haemorrhage*—combines features of the above. This is the most common.

Associated factors
- High parity and poor nutrition
- Pre-eclampsia—due to associated placental bed damage
- Sudden reduction in uterine volume, e.g. when a patient with hydramnios loses a large volume of liquor
- External cephalic version (occasionally)
- Trauma (rarely)
- Previous abruption.

MATERNAL RISKS

- *Disseminated intravascular coagulation* (DIC)—see page 163
- *Hypovolaemic shock*—blood loss is often underestimated, particularly if 'concealed'
- *Postpartum haemorrhage* (see p. 159)—associated with DIC or bleeding into myometrium interfering with uterine contraction ('Couvelaire uterus')
- *Renal failure*—acute tubular necrosis may result from hypovolaemia and intravascular coagulation within the kidney
- *Maternal death*—there were three direct deaths from placental abruption in the UK between 1991 and 1993
- *Recurrence*—may be as high as 17% after one and 25% after two previous placental abruptions.

FETAL RISKS

- *IUGR*—due to association with pre-eclampsia syndrome (see p. 60)
- Perinatal death—overall rates are almost meaningless but about 50% of perinatal deaths are stillbirths
- *Perinatal morbidity*—including birth asphyxia—see page 174.

CLINICAL FEATURES OF SEVERE PLACENTAL ABRUPTION

- Intense, constant abdominal pain with or without vaginal bleeding
- A degree of shock out of proportion to extent of blood loss
- Tender uterus perhaps large for dates and increasing in size
- Fetal parts may be difficult to feel
- Fetal heart sounds may be irregular or absent
- Proteinuria
- DIC may develop
- Oliguria or anuria in really severe cases

DIFFERENTIAL DIAGNOSIS

Among them are:
- placenta praevia
- uterine rupture
- degeneration of a fibroid
- rectus sheath haematoma
- acute hydramnios
- acute surgical conditions.

MANAGEMENT

- Single episode of slight bleeding, mother and fetus in good condition:
  —before 36 weeks' gestation—manage conservatively (as for placenta praevia) and monitor fetal welfare regularly (see p. 57)
  —induce labour (if indicated) at 38 to 40 weeks.
- Severe abruption:
  —begin resuscitation at home before transfer to hospital
  —admit by ambulance with a trained paramedic crew (accompanied by midwife or GP if possible)
  —correct shock and hypovolaemia with intravenous fluids. Monitor central venous pressure and urine volume
  —expedite delivery by amniotomy and judicious oxytocin
  —monitor FHR continuously—an acidotic (hypoxic) fetus should be delivered by caesarean section
  —a case can be made for caesarean section in some situations in which the fetus is already dead, such as when the cervix is tightly shut and amniotomy is impossible; e.g. there is, as yet, no DIC but if the uterus were not to be emptied quickly the risk of its developing would be high
  —check for DIC
  —*beware of postpartum haemorrhage.* Hysterectomy may be necessary in some rare circumstances. It must neither be carried out too soon nor too late! The judgment of a senior obstetrician is mandatory.

OTHER CAUSES OF ANTEPARTUM HAEMORRHAGE

LOCAL CAUSES

For example:
- vaginitis
- cervical polyp
- cervical ectropion
- carcinoma of cervix.

A gentle speculum examination will help to detect these.

UNKNOWN CAUSE

- Do not ignore antepartum haemorrhage even if its cause cannot be determined. There is a high incidence of pre-term delivery in this group.

- Fetal welfare should be monitored for the remainder of pregnancy with the patient in or out of hospital as clinical circumstances dictate.

POLYHYDRAMNIOS

Definition
An excessive volume of amniotic fluid. It can be chronic or acute: the latter can mimic abruptio placentae.

Associated features
- Maternal diabetes
- Multiple pregnancy (especially monovular twins)
- Fetal anomaly, e.g. neural tube defect, oesophageal atresia
- Hydrops fetalis.

Consequences
- Maternal discomfort
- Unstable lie of the fetus
- Increased incidence of pre-term labour
- If the membranes rupture prematurely the following may happen:
  —prolapsed cord
  —malpresentation of fetus
  —placental abruption.

Management
- Check glucose tolerance in all except minor cases.
- Carry out ultrasound scan and/or abdominal X-ray to screen for fetal anomalies.
- Amniocentesis should be considered in severe cases but it often produces only brief respite and may induce pre-term labour.
- In diabetic women tighter control of the diabetes may cause some lessening of fluid volume.
- Test the infant for oesophageal atresia at birth.

FETAL HYDROPS

Definition
The accumulation of fluid in some or all of the serous cavities in the fetus accompanied by generalised oedema of the skin. The placenta may also be oedematous. Fetal ascites can be an early manifestation.

Causes
Although in 15–30% of cases a cause is not identifiable, among the best recognised causes are:
- Rhesus (anti-D) iso-immunisation—at one time the commonest, now rare (see p. 93). It can also occasionally occur against the

blood group antigens K (Kell), Fya (Duffy) or C and E (Rhesus). This group of cases is *'immune hydrops'*.

The remainder are *'non-immune'* hydrops, e.g.:
- cardiovascular lesions—e.g. many cardiac anomalies, congenital heart block, tachydysrhythmias
- chromosomal disorders—e.g. trisomies (particularly trisomy 21), Turner syndrome, triploidy
- congenital malformations—e.g. several recognised syndromes, diaphragmatic herniae, bladder neck obstruction
- haematological—e.g. β-thalassaemia, glucose-6-phosphate dehydrogenase deficiency
- twin–twin transfusion syndrome
- infections, e.g. parvovirus B19, CMV, toxoplasmosis, rubella, syphilis
- placental and umbilical cord lesions—chorioangioma, feto-maternal transfusion, umbilical vein thrombosis
- maternal conditions—severe diabetes or anaemia, hypoproteinaemia.

Incidence
- 'Immune' fetal hydrops affects 2–3% of women with anti-D or other antibodies.
- The ratio of 'non-immune' to 'immune' causes is about 9:1.
- The incidence of 'non-immune' hydrops is about 1/1000 pregnancies.

Investigation
- Antenatal detection is possible in most cases.
- Ultrasound is the most important for initial detection and subsequent assessment.
- Maternal blood—blood group and antibodies; and to exclude G-6-PD deficiency, β-thalassaemia, infection and Kleihauer test.
- Fetal heart monitoring and echocardiography may be helpful.
- Amniocentesis—karyotype; amniotic fluid AFP, CMV culture, and specific metabolic tests.
- Cordocentesis (see p. 51)—fetal blood for IgM, karyotype, DNA analysis and metabolic tests as indicated.

Management
Depends on the cause and severity of the condition.
- Those presenting before 24 weeks tend to have a worse prognosis than those presenting later.
- Currently the only cases amenable to fetal therapy (see p. 52) are those due to poor cardiac output (e.g. anaemia, tachydysrhythmias, hydrothorax, 'twin–twin' transfusion syndrome). This includes only about 20–30% of cases.

MALPRESENTATIONS
HIGH HEAD AT TERM

- Though not strictly a malpresentation it may develop into one during labour.
- It is common in multiparous patients, and in one third of all primigravidae the head remains unengaged at term.
- Among the potential causes to be considered particularly in primigravidae are:
  —greater than average angle of inclination of the brim, e.g. in black women
  —a deflexed head
  —head too large to enter pelvis easily—hydrocephalus; large baby
  —pelvis too small
  —something in the way—placenta praevia, fibroid, the head of an undiagnosed twin
  —too much room for movement, e.g. hydramnios.
- If a significant cause can be ruled out there is no cause for concern.

VARIABLE LIE TOWARDS TERM

- If the fetal lie is persistently variable from 37 weeks' gestation admission is advised lest labour begins and/or the membranes rupture with the fetal lie other than longitudinal.
- Exclude causes such as wrong dates, placenta praevia, multiple pregnancy, and pelvic tumour.
- If the lie stabilises to longitudinal, the mother can be allowed home.
- If the variable lie persists to 41 weeks consider elective caesarean section. However, many women are unwilling to wait that long so each case must be considered individually.

BREECH PRESENTATION (see p. 146).

FACE AND BROW PRESENTATION (see p. 150).

MULTIPLE PREGNANCY

- The incidence of monozygous twinning is 3.5/1000 births.
- Dizygous twinning rates vary widely because they are influenced by maternal age, parity, ethnicity and assisted conception. There is also a familial tendency.
- The incidence of triplets is about $1:80^2$ and of quadruplets about $1:80^3$.
- Histological confirmation of zygosity is necessary after delivery.

Clinical features
- Regular antenatal clinic attendance is advised because all the

hazards of pregnancy are increased, particularly miscarriage, anaemia, pre-eclampsia, hydramnios, pre-term labour and intrapartum problems:
—major congenital malformations are twice as common as in singleton pregnancies
—iron and folic acid supplements are advised
—10% of all pre-term labours are associated with multiple pregnancy
—prophylactic oral tocolytic drugs do not reduce the risk of pre-term labour.
- Routine admission for rest has not been shown to prolong pregnancy.
- Admit if any complications supervene (e.g. pre-eclampsia) or the cervix is effacing too soon.
- Carry out serial checks of fetal growth and welfare (see p. 57).
- Intrauterine death of one twin can occur and the risk of harm or death of the surviving twin is increased thereafter (particularly in monozygous twins).

PROBLEMS WITH MONOZYGOUS TWINS

- In *monochorial, diamniotic twins* (about 70% of twins) placental vascular anastomosis can cause *twin–twin transfusion syndrome* resulting in problems outlined in the box.

Receiving twin	Donor twin
• polycythaemia	• anaemia
• acute, severe polyhydramnios (usually in the second trimester)	• severe oligo- or anhydramnios— the fetus seems to be fixed to uterine side wall—a 'stuck twin'
• fetal hydrops	• IUGR

—without intervention the risk of pre-term delivery is high and fetal outlook is poor
—diagnosis and management depend on detailed ultrasonography and expertise most likely to be found in a recognised Fetal Medicine Unit
—therapeutic amniocentesis is likely to be necessary. For more detailed management see 'High Risk Pregnancy' in Further Reading.
- In *monochorial, monomniotic twins* (about 1% of twins) the placental circulations anastomose completely and the umbilical cords may become intertwined.
—this can lead to *cord entanglement*, occlusion and fetal death— the risk seems to be greater before 30 weeks so elective pre-term delivery may not be indicated

—*conjoint twins* comprise 1% of monozygotic twins. The extent of the conjunction is variable

—*twin reversed arterial perfusion (TRAP) sequence* is a rare complication (about 1/35 000 births). It results from arterial anastomosis allowing competition between the two circulations early in pregnancy. It produces multiple major anomalies in one twin (the so-called 'acardiac monster'). The extra load on the 'pump' twin may cause heart failure with hydrops and polyhydramnios. Pre-term delivery is likely (see Further Reading).

POST-TERM PREGNANCY

- A pregnancy is post-term when it extends beyond 293 days (42 weeks) from the first day of the last menstrual period (LMP).
- The risk of perinatal death is low (2.4/1000 for normally formed babies) in post-term pregnancy.
- There is no reliable evidence to suggest that routine fetal surveillance (see p. 57) will detect those at particular risk (see CPCD in Further Reading).
- Meta-analysis of trials of elective induction of labour for post-term pregnancy (see CPCD) suggests that:
  —such a policy is 'not associated with any major disadvantage'
  —may reduce the already small risk of perinatal death
  —does not affect vaginal operative delivery rates while slightly reducing the risk of delivery by caesarean section.
- The mother should be allowed to make an informed choice about induction of labour.

FURTHER READING

Chamberlain G (ed) 1995 Turnbull's obstetrics. Churchill Livingstone, Edinburgh

The Cochrane Collaboration 1995 Cochrane Pregnancy and Childbirth Database. BMJ Publications, London

Creasy R K, Resnik R (eds) 1994 Maternal–fetal medicine—principles and practice. Saunders, Philadelphia

James D K, Steer P J, Weiner C P, Gonik B 1994 High risk pregnancy—management options. Saunders, London

MacGillivray I, Campbell D M, Thompson B (eds) 1988 Twinning and twins. Wiley, Chichester

10. Labour and intrapartum problems

PHYSIOLOGY OF PARTURITION

Uterine growth is stimulated by mechanical stretching and oestrogens. New muscle forms only in early pregnancy; hypertrophy occurs in mid-pregnancy and distension thereafter.

Uterine activity before labour. Uterine muscle contracts rhythmically even when isolated.

- As they contract, myometrial fibres also retract (i.e. they preserve the same tone but shorten). This is the mechanism by which the physiological lower segment forms late in pregnancy and cervical dilatation occurs during labour.
- Progesterone blocks myometrial excitability; sensitivity to oxytocin increases as pregnancy advances; responses to prostaglandins (PGs) are the same throughout.
- Uterine contractions during the first 20 weeks are of high frequency but low intensity. Frequency and amplitude increase thereafter. Irregular, low-frequency, high-amplitude (Braxton–Hicks) contractions are most apparent in the last 2 months.
- As labour approaches the activity of the fundal myometrium increases most while the lower segment remains relatively inactive. The cervix thus becomes effaced, and engagement of the presenting part is encouraged.

INITIATION OF LABOUR

Maternal and feto-placental factors are involved in the onset of spontaneous labour.

MATERNAL FACTORS

- *Myometrium* remains relatively quiescent despite massive stretching due to the action of progesterone.
- Removal of this block (see below) may facilitate the onset of labour. PGs are involved locally in the action of the myometrial cell but are probably not the primary stimulus.
- *Decidua* is a prime source of PGs.
- The *posterior pituitary gland* produces oxytocin but there is no increase in levels before the onset of labour.

FETO-PLACENTAL FACTORS

- *The placenta*—in many animals progesterone levels fall as oestrogens rise near the onset of labour. Oestrogen stimulates PG production (see below) and the fall in progesterone increases myometrial excitability. The change in the oestrogen/progesterone ratio is much less in humans and no direct relationship between changes and the onset of labour has been shown.
- *Fetal membranes*—the amnion is a potent source of PGs.
- *Fetal pituitary adrenal axis*:
  —throughout most of fetal life the main products of the fetal anterior pituitary are the peptide fragments of adrenocorticotrophic hormone (ACTH) known as α-MSH (α-melanotrophin) and CLIP (corticotrophin-like intermediate lobe peptide) which drive the fetal zone of the adrenal
  —a switch occurs to intact ACTH near term which stimulates development of the definitive adrenal cortex. The production of cortisol by ACTH is important in the initiation of labour in several species (e.g. sheep) but is not essential in man
  —prolactin is the second trophic agent for the fetal adrenal and it encourages oestrogen production.

POSSIBLE SEQUENCE OF EVENTS

- Progesterone-binding protein increases at term: the tissue effects of progesterone decrease.
- The suppression of myometrial excitability by progesterone decreases.
- The relative fall in progesterone also promotes the release of arachidonic acid.
- ACTH promotes production of dehydroepiandrosterone (DHEA) in the fetal adrenal which goes on to form oestrone and oestradiol.
- Oestrogens further stimulate the production of arachidonic acid.
- PGs are produced in decidua and fetal membranes.
- Labour is initiated.

NORMAL LABOUR

Normal labour is characterised by:
- regular uterine contractions
- dilatation of the cervix
- descent of the presenting part.

It encompasses the time from the onset of regular contractions to spontaneous vaginal delivery of the infant (within 24 hours).

UTERINE CONTRACTIONS

- Contractions begin in two 'pace-makers' near the uterotubal junctions.

- Only one is operative in each contraction, which spreads like a wave over the whole uterus.
- Relaxation begins simultaneously in all areas of the uterus.
- Labour is characterised by:
  —strong and sustained action of the muscle of the uterine fundus which increases as labour progresses
  —less strong contractions of the mid-zone
  —relative inactivity of the lower segment.
- Normal uterine contractions are characterised by:
  —a frequency of one every 2–3 minutes with at least 1 minute between contractions
  —a duration of 40–70 seconds
  —an intensity (measured by intrauterine catheter) of around 50 mmHg with a resting tonus of <10 mmHg.

CERVICAL DILATATION

- This occurs from above downwards accompanied by effacement (thinning).
- It is caused by coordinated contraction and retraction of the upper segment.
- The forewaters may act as a hydrostatic wedge, and dilatation is facilitated by close apposition of the cervix and presenting part.

FIRST STAGE OF LABOUR

Latent and active phases—see Table 10.1.
- The latent phase starts from the onset of regular uterine contractions and ends when the cervix is 2–3 cm dilated and fully effaced. It occurs because the thinning of the lower segment and cervix take a lot of uterine work before rapid dilatation can begin.
- In the active phase the cervix dilates at 1–3 cm per hour in primigravidae and up to 6 cm per hour in multigravidae.

Table 10.1 Length of first stage of labour

| | Mean length in hours (± 1SD) | |
	Primigravidae	Multigravidae
Latent phase	9 ± 6	5 ± 4
Active phase	5 ± 3.5	2 ± 1.5

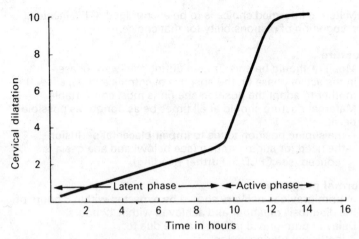

Fig 10.1 Cervical dilatation time curve

Control of uterine activity in labour
- PGs are, and oxytocin may be, important for the maintenance of progressive labour.
- The autonomic nervous system has little or no motor function.

Progress in labour
Best assessed using a *partogram* on which can be recorded:
- cervical dilatation—marked in centimetres at zero time (the time of admission to labour ward) and at every subsequent examination
- descent of the head (in fifths palpable above the pelvic brim)
- contractions—frequency, duration and strength assessed for 10 minutes each half-hour
- fetal heart rate (see p. 142)
- condition of the liquor, and time and manner of membrane rupture
- moulding of the fetal skull
- dosage of oxytocin, if used
- maternal status (BP, pulse, temperature, urinalysis) and medication (including epidural block, if used).

MANAGEMENT OF NORMAL LABOUR
- Each obstetric unit should set down (and review regularly) agreed guidelines for the management of labour to include a clear statement about the diagnosis of the onset of labour.
- Routine perineal shaving and an enema on admission are outmoded practices.

- Maternal informed choice is to be encouraged. (This includes recognition of responsibility for that choice.)

Posture
- Mobility should be encouraged during the latent phase.
- In the active phase (in the absence of complications), allow the mother to adopt the position she finds most comfortable.
- Maternal posture should at all times be as upright as possible because:
  —the supine position tends to impair placental perfusion
  —the need for augmentation (see below) and analgesia is reduced (see CPCD in Further Reading).

Normal progress
- In primigravidae delivery should be expected within 8 hours of the diagnosis of labour and achieved within 12 hours.
- Delay in primigravid labour may be due to:
  —inefficient uterine action
  —occipito-posterior position of the fetal head
  —true cephalo-pelvic disproportion (rarely).
- Labour is much more rapid in multiparous women, and inefficient uterine action is rare. *If delay is occurring its cause should be sought and corrected if possible.*
- Obstruction must be considered as a possible cause for prolonged labour in a multiparous woman.

AUGMENTATION OF LABOUR IN PRIMIGRAVIDAE

- This practice remains controversial. Its aim is to achieve safe delivery within 8 hours of admission to the labour ward.
- It is usually considered if the rate of cervical dilatation is less than 1 cm per hour in the active phase of labour.
- The membranes are ruptured and oxytocin infusion is set up 1 hour later if labour does not accelerate.
- Among the contraindications are:
  —obstetric anomalies, e.g. breech presentation or multiple pregnancy
  —fetal compromise.
- *It is relatively contraindicated in multigravidae because the risk of uterine rupture is high.*
- Review of trials to date (see CPCD in Further Reading) suggests that:
  —no beneficial effects have been demonstrated
  —women find ambulation more acceptable
  —further trials are necessary.

ORAL INTAKE IN LABOUR

- The major risk to be avoided is aspiration of gastric contents. This only occurs in the context of general anaesthesia.

- In general therefore, low-fat, low-residue food and drink can be given to a mother during labour.
- There is no evidence that the routine use of antacids or H$_2$-receptor antagonists is beneficial.
- The significance of *ketonuria* is exaggerated:
  —intravenous infusions of dextrose solutions (particularly dextrose 10%) are contraindicated because of their deleterious effect on mother and baby
  —if dehydration needs to be corrected, normal saline should be infused but *the volume must not exceed 3 litres/24 hours*.

SECOND STAGE OF LABOUR

- It begins with full dilatation of the cervix and ends with delivery of the baby.
- Its average length in primigravidae is 40 minutes, and in multiparae is 20 minutes.
- It has two phases:
  —the *propulsive phase* from full dilatation until the presenting part has descended to the pelvic floor
  —the *expulsive phase* which ends with delivery of the baby and is recognised by the mother's irresistible desire to bear down and/or distension of the perineum.
- A woman should not usually be encouraged to bear down until she has entered the expulsive phase.
- A prolonged propulsive phase in primigravidae due to inefficient uterine action (and not cephalo-pelvic disproportion) can be treated judiciously with oxytocin.

INDUCTION OF LABOUR

- Induction of labour can be justified when:
  —the intrauterine risks to the fetus outweigh those from delivery
  —the risk to the mother's health from the continuation of pregnancy outweighs the risk to the fetus from delivery.
- If the added risk of labour is unacceptable, delivery must be by caesarean section.
- Otherwise, labour can be induced and the maternal and fetal state monitored throughout.
- The optimum time for delivery is often difficult to judge, and secure knowledge of gestational age is important.
- 'Social' indications rarely constitute an adequate reason for induction but each situation must be considered on its merits.

CONTRAINDICATIONS

Absolute
- The fetal lie is not longitudinal.

- Caesarean section has been carried out in a previous pregnancy for a recurrent reason, e.g. pelvic contraction.
- Two previous caesarean sections have been performed.
- A tumour occupies the pelvis.

Relative
- The cervix has previously been repaired. Previous cone biopsy merits caution.
- Highly multiparous woman.

Other factors to be borne in mind
- An unfavourable cervix.
- Uncertain gestational age.

HAZARDS

- *Iatrogenic prematurity*—early pregnancy dating by ultrasound reduces this risk.
- *Infection*—there is little appreciable risk in practice but amnionitis can always be detected within 36 hours of amniotomy.
- *Neonatal jaundice*—there is a small risk if the total dose of oxytocin exceeds 20 units.
- *Failed induction*—defined as failure to deliver vaginally a patient in whom safe vaginal delivery was expected. The incidence is about 2% of all inductions.
- Additional hazards—induced labours are longer, require more analgesia, have a higher incidence of instrumental delivery and caesarean section, and lower Apgar scores than comparable spontaneous labours.

CERVICAL RIPENESS

- This is assessed by a 'Bishop score' which gives marks of 0–3 for five cervical features:
  —dilatation (cm)　　　　　—consistency
  —length (cm)　　　　　　—position
  —station of head
  　(cm above ischial spines)
- If the cervix is 'ripe' (score >5) induction of labour is likely to be successful.
- With a score of <5 induction is more likely to fail, the latent phase will tend to be longer, and a higher total dose of oxytocin will be necessary to reach optimal uterine activity.
- The cervix can be ripened with vaginal prostaglandin E_2 (the dose is less for multiparous than primigravid women). Hyperstimulation of the uterus is rare but can occur. Frequent low-amplitude contractions within 20 minutes of insertion are common.

- Fetal heart rate monitoring is advisable if induction is being carried out for fetal reasons.

METHODS OF INDUCTION

- Vaginal prostaglandin may induce labour, particularly in women with a favourable cervix.
- Amniotomy.
- Oxytocin infusion by peristaltic or syringe pump:
  —the dose of oxytocin required to produce effective uterine action is between 4 and 16 milliunits per minute (mu/min). Occasionally as much as 32 mu/min are necessary
  —as labour becomes established the uterus becomes more sensitive to oxytocin and the effective dose rate reduces to about 8 mu/min.
- Actual regimes are numerous but each must follow the following principles:
  —low doses initially, gradually increasing to produce effective contractions
  —dose rate varied to suit the individual woman
  —any complications such as hyperstimulation must be detected early.
- Water intoxication has occasionally followed the infusion of large volumes of oxytocin-containing fluid. Confusion and convulsions can proceed to coma and even death. *This is totally avoidable.*
- For more detailed discussion see Further Reading.

PAIN IN LABOUR

Pain is a normal part of labour and delivery, although emotional, cultural and other influences alter individual responses.

Causes of pain in labour
- Dilatation of the cervix
- Contraction and distension of the uterus, possibly due to the accumulation of pain-producing substances during ischaemia
- Distension of vagina and perineum
- Pressure on other organs (e.g. bladder and rectum) or the lumbosacral plexus; spasm in skeletal muscles.

Sensory pathways are T10 to L1 for both uterine body and cervix. T11 and 12 are stimulated during latent phase when pain is not severe, T10–L1 are stimulated during the active phase. Referred pain is experienced in the dermatomes of the above segments.

Factors affecting pain in childbirth
- Physical factors including:
  —intensity and duration of contractions

—speed of dilatation of cervix
—vaginal and perineal distension
—other factors, e.g. age, parity, size of infant, condition of patient.
- Physiological factors:
  —pain blocking, e.g. customs, culture, preparation, distractive activity
  —pain aggravating, e.g. customs, culture, fear, apprehension, anxiety, ignorance, misinformation.
- Antenatal preparation of the mother and father are very important.

ANALGESIA

Antenatal education is a vital part of preparing women for the pain of labour.

METHODS FOR PAIN RELIEF

Psychological methods
- Counteract the 'fear–tension' sequence.
- Pain-relieving drugs can be used to supplement the mother's own efforts.
- With proper training, 30–40% of women can go through labour without requiring analgesic drugs.

Inhalational agents
- Nitrous oxide (50%) and oxygen (50%)—'Entonox' apparatus
- Inhalational agents are usually used too late and too hesitantly
- They can be highly effective and safe for mother and baby.

Transcutaneous electrical nerve stimulation (TENS)
- This aims to reduce pain by stimulating large myelinated nerve fibres to reduce input from small myelinated and non-myelinated fibres linked to peripheral pain receptors.
- Low-intensity continuous stimulation is applied to the dermatomes associated with the pain.
- It can provide good to moderate pain relief but success depends on time spent teaching and supporting the mother before and during use.

Narcotic drugs
- E.g. intramuscular pethidine
- Combination with a phenothiazine (e.g. promazine or promethazine) provides no additional benefit, may produce maternal and fetal tachycardia and can rarely cause an oculogyric crisis.

Advantages
- Ease of administration

- Reasonably rapid analgesia
- Low incidence of serious side-effects
- Antagonists available.

Disadvantages
- Inadequate analgesia in up to 40% of patients
- Nausea and vomiting common
- Psychic disturbances common, e.g. confusion, inability to cooperate
- Delayed gastric emptying
- Neonatal respiratory depression.

Contraindications
- Previous idiosyncratic reactions
- Current monoamine oxidase inhibitors.

Epidural analgesia
- Despite its widespread use, little is known about the short- or long-term effects of epidural block on mother or baby (see CPCD in Further Reading).
- Lumbar analgesia will provide total or adequate analgesia in up to 90% of patients.

Indications If epidural analgesia is not available on request it may be helpful for:
- prolonged labour
- maternal distress
- multiple pregnancy
- instrumental delivery
- hypertension in labour
- breech presentation?

Contraindications
- lack of experienced personnel
- infection at the injection site
- coagulation defects or bleeding diathesis
- idiosyncratic reactions to local anaesthetic agents
- shock and hypovolaemia
- bony abnormalities of the spinal column
- anticoagulant therapy

Pre-existing neurological disease is not necessarily a contraindication as long as it is understood that coincidental relapses can occur unrelated to the epidural block.

Immediate maternal problems
- *Dural tap*—dural puncture by needle or catheter; it leads to 'spinal' headache (see below)
- *Total spinal block*—loss of all sensory and motor function; can include unconsciousness, severe hypotension and apnoea; results from subarachnoid injection of epidural dose of local anaesthetic agent

- *Hypotension*—can be avoided by nursing the patient on her side and by the intravenous infusion of Hartmann's solution before the block is established (also used for treatment of hypotension)
- *Motor paralysis*—reduces maternal expulsive effort, tends to prevent rotation of the fetal head and makes instrumental delivery more likely. Risk of caesarean section may also be raised
- *Prolongation of second stage* of labour
- *Toxic reactions* to local anaesthetic agents.

Delayed maternal hazards
- Severe *spinal headache* due to spinal tap (infuse 1 litre of normal saline through the epidural catheter over 24 h; if no improvement within 48 hours consider a 'blood patch' (i.e. injection of up to 20 ml autologous blood into epidural space)
- *Urinary retention*—? more usually due to method and circumstances of delivery
- *Sepsis*—extremely unlikely if bacterial filter is used
- *Temporary diminished sensation* of dermatomes affected
- *Backache* is an occasional problem.

Fetal effects
There are no direct adverse effects on the fetus.

Guidelines for use
- The regional block may be continuous during labour or as a single injection for operative delivery.
- Bupivacaine (0.5, 0.375 or 0.25%) is the preferred anaesthetic—a test dose should be injected initially.
- Constant monitoring of maternal and fetal condition is mandatory.
- Top-up dose must be individually chosen when the patient begins to experience discomfort.

Epidural analgesia and previous caesarean section
Epidural block is permissible in any woman who is being allowed to labour having previously been delivered by caesarean section. FHR and ideally intrauterine pressure should be monitored throughout.

PRE-TERM LABOUR AND DELIVERY

Definition
Regular, painful uterine contractions accompanied by effacement and dilatation of the cervix after 20 and before 37 completed weeks of pregnancy. It accounts for 5–10% of all deliveries but 85% of neonatal deaths.

FACTORS ASSOCIATED WITH PRE-TERM DELIVERY

- Spontaneous labour—cause unknown: 40%
- Spontaneous labour due to maternal or fetal conditions other than multiple pregnancy: 25%
- Multiple pregnancy: 10%
- Elective delivery: 25%.

CAUSES OF SPONTANEOUS PRE-TERM LABOUR

These are given in the box (roughly in order of importance).

Spontaneous pre-term labour: causes	
• Multiple pregnancy	• Congenital uterine anomaly
• Antepartum haemorrhage	• Diabetes
• Intrauterine growth retardation	• Polyhydramnios
• Cervical incompetence	• Pyelonephritis
• Amnionitis	• Other infections

PREDICTION OF RISK

- No scoring system yet devised has proven itself superior to clinical judgment.
- The strongest association is with previous pre-term delivery.
- Among the measures suggested for prediction of high risk and possible prevention and for which no evidence of benefit exists are:
  —routine cervical examination
  —home monitoring of uterine activity
  —prophylactic β-sympathomimetics
  —routine screening for bacterial vaginosis
  —prophylactic antibiotics.
- It has, however, recently been suggested (see Iams et al 1996 in Further Reading) that the risk tends to increase, the shorter the cervix measured by vaginal ultrasound at about 24 and 28 weeks. The information box outlines statistics.

Length of cervix (at or below percentile)	Length of cervix (mm)	Relative risk of pre-term delivery
75th	40	2
10th	26	6
5th	22	9.5
1st	13	14

MANAGEMENT VARIES ACCORDING TO FIVE MAIN FACTORS

- *The state of the membranes*—the efficacy or even advisability of attempts to inhibit pre-term labour when the membranes are ruptured is open to question.
- *Dilatation of the cervix*—labour is likely to progress if the cervix is >4 cm dilated.
- *Gestational age*—the earlier the gestation, the more strenuous attempts to inhibit labour must be. Labour should be allowed to progress if the estimated fetal weight is >2000 g.
- *The cause of pre-term labour*—delivery is indicated if fetal welfare is prejudiced:
  —carry out an infection screen on the mother and consider amniocentesis for bacteriological culture
  —assess fetal well-being (see p. 57).
- *The availability of neonatal intensive care facilities*—if all cots are full or facilities are inadequate, consider transfer of the patient (in good time) to a unit with better facilities.

GLUCOCORTICOID THERAPY AND THE PREVENTION OF RESPIRATORY DISTRESS SYNDROME

- Corticosteroids given to the mother between 24 and 34 weeks can induce pulmonary surfactant in the lungs of the immature fetus.
- One regimen is dexamethasone 12 mg i.m. on 2 successive days repeated 2-weekly to 34 weeks.

INHIBITION OF PRE-TERM LABOUR

- In up to 50% of patients contractions will stop spontaneously and the pregnancy will continue to term without any treatment whatsoever.
- The clinical problem is to discern correctly those in whom drug therapy is indicated.

β-sympathomimetic drugs
- These drugs, e.g. salbutamol or ritodrine hydrochloride, suppress uterine activity.
- Prolongation of pregnancy is, however, not necessarily beneficial to the fetus.
- *The only true indication for their use is to delay delivery* for long enough to allow:
  —glucocorticoids to stimulate fetal lung surfactant (see above)
  —transfer of the mother to a centre with adequate facilities for pre-term delivery.

- Potential side-effects:
  - —maternal tachycardia
  - —hypotension
  - —palpitations, headache, visual disturbances, skin flushing, nausea and vomiting
  - —fetal tachycardia
  - —hyperkalaemia
  - —hyperglycaemia
  - —rarely right heart failure may develop (usually when glucocorticoids have also been given).

Contraindications
- Antepartum haemorrhage
- Severe pre-eclampsia
- Maternal anti-hypertensive therapy (risk of myocardial infarction)
- Maternal cardiac disease or thyrotoxicosis
- Any other situation in which the prolongation of pregnancy could be hazardous
- Extreme caution must be exercised if the woman has diabetes, or is being treated with corticosteroids.

METHOD OF DELIVERY IN PRE-TERM LABOUR

- If the fetus is viable it must be delivered by the route least likely to cause trauma or hypoxia.
- Aim to have an experienced neonatal paediatrician present for delivery.
- In general, aim for vaginal delivery if gestation <26 weeks.
- Caesarean sections at early gestation, and with infants under 1000 g, can be hazardous for the mother and are not necessarily safer for the baby.
- The indications for caesarean section are stronger but not absolute in multiple pregnancy and breech presentation.
- Pre-term labour is unpredictable and the woman may become fully dilated quickly and silently.

PREMATURE RUPTURE OF THE MEMBRANES (PROM)

Definition
Rupture of the membranes before the onset of labour without reference to gestational age.
- It can be managed conservatively before 34–36 weeks' gestation unless intrauterine infection is present or likely to develop.
- A high vaginal swab should be taken on admission. If it grows any significant organisms (particularly β-haemolytic streptococci), delivery should be expedited and the neonatal paediatricians alerted. Any intrauterine infection must be treated vigorously and expeditiously.
- In term pregnancies 90% of women with PROM go into labour within 24 hours and deliver satisfactorily. In the absence of any evidence of infection or cord presentation/prolapse, the onset of

labour can be awaited for 24 (and possibly 48) hours. Labour can be induced in those women who remain undelivered.

INTRAPARTUM FETAL MONITORING

- The aim is to detect fetal hypoxia.
- The effects of hypoxia depend on the fetal glycogen reserves. A growth-retarded fetus will therefore be affected earlier and more severely than a well-nourished fetus:
  —anaerobic glycolysis results in an accumulation of lactate. This causes a fetal metabolic acidosis
  —the fetal PCO_2 rises, causing a respiratory acidosis
  —the blood pH falls
  —fetal heart rate patterns change (see below), the most serious being decelerations.
- The traditional diagnosis of 'fetal distress' depended predominantly on the crude observation of heart changes.
- 'Fetal distress' is an imprecise and rather unhelpful term. Half of all babies delivered by forceps or caesarean section because of 'fetal distress' are not hypoxic; and half of the most hypoxic babies do not exhibit classical signs of 'fetal distress'.

METHODS OF INTRAPARTUM MONITORING

Intermittent recording of fetal heart rate (FHR) using a fetal stethoscope:

- between contractions to obtain a baseline rate
- during and immediately after contractions to detect accelerations or decelerations
- applicable only to low-risk patients with no obstetric abnormalities
- more intensive monitoring should be used if any risk factors are present (see below).

CONTINUOUS RECORDING OF FHR AND UTERINE ACTIVITY (CARDIOTOCOGRAPHY—CTG)

- The FHR is best obtained by an electrode attached to fetal scalp (or buttock).
- The monitor measures the interval between paired beats, converts it into 'beats per minute' (b.p.m) and registers it.
- Uterine activity can be assessed by an external strain gauge transducer or measured by intrauterine catheter.
- *This is a screening technique which facilitates the detection of fetal hypoxic stress.* It is not diagnostic.
- Even when the most ominous pattern is present (see below) only 50% of the babies have a low Apgar score (see p. 174) at birth.
- The use of continuous FHR recordings must therefore be backed up by measurement of fetal scalp pH (see over).

Guide to indications for continuous FHR monitoring in labour

Antepartum risk factors:
- primigravidae aged 35 or over; multigravidae aged 40 or over
- high multiparity
- suspected IUGR
- pregnancy-induced hypertension
- history of APH in this pregnancy
- bad obstetric history

- diabetes
- multiple pregnancy
- Rhesus iso-immunisation
- oligohydramnios
- reduced fetal movements
- abnormal antenatal FHR tracing.

Intrapartum risk factors:
- FHR >160 or <120 b.p.m.
- meconium-stained liquor
- prolonged labour
- epidural anaesthesia

- augmented labour
- pre-term labour
- breech presentation
- supine hypotension.

Interpretation. The whole clinical situation must be considered.

Normal pattern
- Rate between 120 and 160 b.p.m. observed over at least a 5–10 minute period
- Baseline irregularity/variability of ≥5 b.p.m.
- No significant change in rate during contractions.

Loss of baseline irregularity (<5 b.p.m.)
- The feature most commonly associated with fetal hypoxia
- Maternal drug administration can also reduce it
- Management: check fetal pH.

Baseline bradycardia (FHR <120 b.p.m.)
- Only significant if it is accompanied by loss of baseline irregularity and/or decelerations (i.e. complicated bradycardia)
- Management: turn the patient on her side, give oxygen and check fetal pH.

Baseline tachycardia (FHR >160 b.p.m.)
- Management: measure fetal pH if tachycardia persists or it is accompanied by decelerations and/or loss of baseline irregularity.

Accelerations (at the start of a contraction returning to baseline). This is normal.

Early decelerations ('Type 1 dip')
- A deceleration beginning with the onset of the contraction, returning to the baseline rate by the end of the contraction and usually <40 b.p.m.

- May be due to head compression, cord compression or early hypoxia
- Management: check fetal pH if the pattern deteriorates.

Variable decelerations
- A deceleration appearing at a variable time during the contraction, of irregular shape and >50 b.p.m.
- If they appear consistently, fetal hypoxia is likely
- Management: check fetal pH if the pattern persists after turning the patient on her side (or if other adverse features are present).

Late decelerations
- A deceleration the lowest point of which is past the peak of the contraction
- The greater the lag time the more serious the significance
- The worst picture is of shallow late decelerations, loss of baseline irregularity and tachycardia
- Management: a fetal pH measurement is mandatory.

FHR in the second stage of labour
- The fetal heart patterns are complex and difficult to interpret in the second stage of labour.
- Brief profound decelerations are not uncommon but prolonged bradycardia must not be ignored.

FETAL ECG

- Uses the same scalp clip as for the FHR
- Depends on analysis of the ST waveform
- The following adverse features have been suggested:
  —T/QRS ratio >0.25
  —a negative T wave
  —ST depression with T elevation
- Main benefit is to provide reassurance in the presence of an abnormal CTG and, perhaps, reduce the rate of unnecessary caesarean sections.

FETAL BLOOD SAMPLING (FBS)

- FHR and scalp pH measurement are complementary.
- The former without the latter increases the caesarean section rate unnecessarily because of false-positive diagnoses.
- The indications for FBS are outlined above.
- A fetal scalp pH of 7 or less is strongly associated with a poor outcome (particularly if the Apgar score is 3 or under at 5 minutes).
- A pH of 7.15 or less suggests the need to deliver.
- A base deficit of >9 mmol/L is also abnormal.

Significance of meconium staining of the liquor

- Meconium is present in the liquor of about 15% of all deliveries at term and up to 40% post-term.
- Its significance as a diagnostic sign of 'fetal distress' has been over-emphasised although gross staining is more likely to be significant.
- Aspiration by the baby of the liquor heavily stained with meconium causes a severe and sometimes fatal pneumonitis. This should therefore be avoided.

Conclusion

The sensitivity and specificity of all methods for intrapartum monitoring of the fetus are still poor. New initiatives are still badly needed. For further discussion see CPCD in Further Reading.

THE NORMAL PELVIS

AVERAGE DIAMETERS

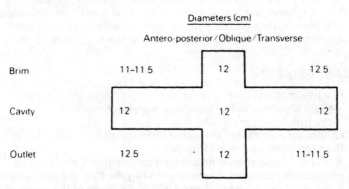

Fig 10.2 The normal pelvis—average diameters

PELVIC SHAPE—IN THE NORMAL PELVIS

- The *brim* is round, and the sacral promontory is not prominent.
- The *angle of inclination* is about 55° to the horizontal.
- The *cavity* is shallow with straight, non-converging walls.
- The *sacrum* is smoothly curved.
- In the *outlet* the sacro-sciatic notches are wide and shallow.
- The *sacrum* does not project forwards.
- The *ischial spines* are not prominent.
- The *public arch* is wide and domed.
- The *sub-pubic angle* is about 90°.
- The *inter-tuberous diameter* is wide.

PELVIMETRY

- Clinical assessment of pelvic size and shape is only likely to be of benefit if the pelvis is severely contracted. ·
- X-ray pelvimetry has been superseded in many places by CT scanning. This reduces the radiation dosage and is likely to be more accurate.
- However, the criteria for normality have not yet been set.
- Pelvimetry is of no clinical value if the presentation is cephalic.
- There is also no reliable evidence of benefit for the traditional indications of primigravid breech presentation or after caesarean section for suspected disproportion.

CEPHALO-PELVIC DISPROPORTION (CPD)

Definition
The failure of the head to pass through the pelvis safely because the pelvis is too small and/or the head too large.
- CPD is more likely if maternal height is 1.5 metres or less.
- The diagnosis is made *in labour* if the fetal head fails to descend and the cervix to dilate. With increasing oedema of the scalp, *caput* forms and excessive moulding of the skull bones occurs.

MANAGEMENT

- Elective section is rarely necessary in primigravidae unless:
  —there are other indications, e.g. a malpresentation
  —the true.conjugate is <7.5 cm.
- Otherwise an attempt at vaginal delivery is justifiable. This is then regarded as a *trial of labour*.
- A trial of labour should be allowed to continue for as long as progress is occurring in labour with regular forceful contractions.
- If the woman has not delivered within 12 hours of the onset of regular contractions the situation must be reviewed critically.
- *Such a trial of labour has no place in multigravid women or in the presence of a breech presentation.*

ABNORMALITIES OF LIE, PRESENTATION AND POSITION

BREECH PRESENTATION

Incidence
2–3% of all labours. Up to one third are undiagnosed.

Definition
- Frank breech (65%)—both legs extended at the knee
- Complete breech (10%)—both legs flexed at hip and knee
- Footling breech (25%)—one or both feet tucked underneath the

buttocks; more common in multiparous women due to laxity of abdomen.

Causes
- Extended legs preventing spontaneous version
- Those conditions preventing the presenting part entering the pelvic cavity
- Uterine anomaly
- Chance.

Associations
- Fetal anomaly
- Pre-term delivery
- Multiple pregnancy.

Antenatal management
- Spontaneous version is likely up to 34 weeks.
- External cephalic version (ECV) is safe for mother and baby in carefully selected patients and reduces the need for elective caesarean section.
- ECV is not advised before 36 weeks. Some advocate the use of tocolytic agents but trial evidence is insufficient to draw any conclusions about their use. Do not use in women with heart disease, diabetes or thyroid disease.

Hazards of ECV. See the information box.

Hazards of ECV	
• Pre-term labour	• Cord accident
• Placental abruption	• Uterine rupture (if previous section)

Contraindications to ECV. See the information box.

Contraindications to ECV	
Absolute	*Relative*
• Multiple pregnancy	• Previous caesarean section
• APH	• IUGR
• Ruptured membranes	• Hypertension
• Oligohydramnios	• Rhesus iso-immunisation
• Significant fetal anomaly	• High multiparity
• Caesarean section indicated for other reasons	• Anterior placenta
	• Obesity

Prerequisites for ECV
- Gestation at least 36 weeks
- Recent ultrasound to confirm presentation, normal fetus and adequate liquor volume
- Reactive FHR
- Informed consent of mother
- Facilities for rapid progression to caesarean section, if necessary
- Rh-D-negative women must be given anti-D immunoglobulin (50 μg or more as Kleihauer test dictates).

Management of delivery
- Some argue that breech presentation is indication enough for caesarean section.
- Although vaginal breech delivery as a whole is associated with a higher perinatal mortality and morbidity than caesarean section, these results are biased by the inclusion in the former group of very low birthweight infants for whom caesarean section was not considered, or who delivered precipitately.
- The benefits of routine caesarean section in both term and pre-term delivery have not been clearly demonstrated (see CPCD in Further Reading).
- A more conservative policy is outlined below.

Pre-delivery assessment
- There is no evidence that routine pelvimetry is beneficial. If thought to be necessary use CT pelvimetry (see p. 146).
- Carry out ultrasound assessment of BPD, fetal mass, fetal attitude and flexion/extension of fetal head.
- Major fetal anomalies should have been excluded.

Vaginal delivery
- An attempt at vaginal delivery can be considered with:
  —term pregnancy and fetal weight estimated at 2500 to 3500 g
  —frank breech
  —presumed or demonstrated normal pelvic dimensions
  —no other complications of pregnancy (e.g. pre-eclampsia)
  —normal fetal assessment.
- Epidural anaesthesia can be useful during a breech labour.
- Augmentation of labour with oxytocin is contraindicated.
- The baby should be born by the patient's own efforts with little assistance from the obstetrician (assisted breech delivery).
- Any more active intervention involving breech extraction is contraindicated because the perinatal consequences are so severe.

Caesarean section

Definite indications are listed in the information box.

Caesarean section: definite indications

- Any abnormality of bony pelvis
- Fetal weight estimated at >3.5 kg
- Hyperextension of fetal head
- Previous difficult labour
- IUGR
- Bad obstetric history
- Older primigravidae

- Diabetes
- Severe pre-eclampsia
- Failure to progress in first stage
- Failure of descent of breech in second stage
- Any condition which would apply whatever the presentation, e.g. fetal hypoxia

---

In the following, caesarean section may be indicated and any attempt at vaginal delivery must be clearly justified:
- complete or footling breech
- pre-term labour
- uterine anomaly
- lesser pregnancy complications than those noted above.

OCCIPITO-POSTERIOR POSITION

If the baby's head is partially extended it does not fit into the lower uterine pole well, with the following consequences in labour:
- the membranes rupture early and the cervix is not well apposed to the cervix
- the sinciput reaches the pelvic floor first and therefore rotates to the front, i.e. the occiput is posterior
- the larger occipito-frontal diameter (10 cm) of the head presents, making its passage through the pelvis more difficult
- the first stage of labour is prolonged
- the moment of the forces pushes the head posteriorly causing backache and inducing bearing-down efforts before full dilatation
- the second stage of labour may be prolonged.

The occiput may:
- rotate anteriorly and deliver relatively easily (75%)
- persist posteriorly (POP) and deliver spontaneously if the pelvis is capacious (i.e. face to pubes) or require assisted delivery (5%)
- begin to rotate anteriorly but undergo deep transverse arrest at the level of the ischial spines. Instrumental delivery will be required (20%).

Predisposing factors
- Slight reduction in pelvic inlet
- Large baby.

Diagnosis
- Antenatally—this is inaccurate:
  —the maternal abdomen may be flattened or fetal parts palpable easily on both sides of the midline
  —the head is unengaged and feels larger than usual.
- Intrapartum—by vaginal examination:
  —both fontanelles can be felt more easily
  —moulding and caput may make recognition difficult and palpation of an ear may be necessary for correct positioning.

Management
- Provide adequate analgesia: an epidural anaesthetic is ideal
- Prevent 'maternal distress' and dehydration
- Observe progress in labour carefully
- Monitor fetal welfare
- Relative cephalo-pelvic disproportion may occur
- The criteria for assisted delivery are discussed on page 155.

BROW PRESENTATION

- A brow presentation discovered antenatally may be due to: chance—and may correct itself spontaneously; a swelling in the neck causing extension of the head, e.g. goitre, cystic hygroma; spasm of the sterno-mastoid muscles.
- Suspect a brow presentation in a multiparous woman with delay in the first stage of labour despite good contractions when she has delivered vaginally easily before.

Diagnosis
- Supra-orbital ridges and anterior fontanelle palpable p.v.
- Confirm by ultrasound.

Management
- In early labour a brow presentation may flex to become a vertex or extend further to a face presentation. Both are potentially deliverable vaginally.
- If the brow presentation persists into, or is discovered in, established labour, delivery should be by caesarean section.

FACE PRESENTATION

- A face presentation has the same causes as a brow presentation but causing full extension of the head on the neck.
- In labour anterior rotation of the chin is essential: a mento-posterior position cannot deliver vaginally.

Diagnosis
Palpation of supra-orbital ridges and the alveolar margins (confusion may arise between a face and the breech). X-ray will help to confirm.

Management
An attempt at vaginal delivery should be allowed unless:
- something is obstructing the entry into the pelvis
- the pelvis is too small
- the chin is posterior.

TRANSVERSE AND OBLIQUE LIE

Principal causes are listed in the box.

Transverse and oblique lie: causes	
• High multiparity	• Hydramnios
• Pre-term labour	• Obstructing tumour or placenta praevia
• Multiple pregnancy	
• Uterine anomaly	• Severe pelvic contraction

Antenatal management
See page 125.

Intrapartum management (singleton pregnancy)
- In a neglected shoulder presentation an arm may well be prolapsed and the baby already dead. In these circumstances vaginal decapitation may be possible but only by an experienced operator.
- Otherwise caesarean section with decapitation in utero is less hazardous for the mother.

SHOULDER DYSTOCIA
- This is one of the most frightening obstetric emergencies.
- It occurs when the fetal shoulders fail to negotiate the pelvic inlet.
- The incidence is 0.2–1%?
- Prompt (but not forcible) action is required to prevent fetal morbidity or mortality.

Antenatal risk factors
- Mother's birthweight >90th percentile
- Maternal obesity or massive weight gain

- Diabetes mellitus—can be *despite* seemingly good blood sugar control
- Prolonged pregnancy (beyond 42 completed weeks)
- Previous shoulder dystocia or large baby
- Recognised macrosomia this pregnancy.

Intrapartum risk factors
First stage:
- 'dysfunctional labour'
- secondary arrest after 8 cm.

Second stage:
- midcavity arrest
- need for midcavity instrumental delivery in multiparous woman.

Prediction?
- Consideration of above risk factors predicts less than 20% of cases!!
  —where practised it has not reduced fetal asphyxia or trauma
  —when interpreted too rigidly, many women will have unnecessary interventions.
- Clinical prediction of excessive birthweight is unreliable.
- Ultrasound estimates are inaccurate at upper percentiles.

Risks to the baby?
- Neurological injury—occurs in 1–2/1000 births. It can involve:
  —cervical cord
  —brachial plexus—Erb's palsy (C5,6,7); Klumpke's palsy (C7,8, T1)
  —phrenic nerve
- Hypoxic ischaemic encephalopathy (HIE)—0.5–1/1000 births
- Fractures—clavicle (2–3/1000); humerus (0.2–0.3/1000).

Management
- Recognition and recording of possible risk factors (keep good records!)
- Clear plan of action in guidelines
- Rapid reaction—the midwife has a vital role
- *Immediate response*:
  —summon experienced obstetrician and anaesthetist
  —place woman in 'McRoberts position', i.e. hip joints fully abducted, rotated outwards and flexed with thighs touching maternal abdomen
  —make good-sized episiotomy.
- *Next steps*:
  —suprapubic pressure to try to dislodge anterior shoulder
  —try to rotate fetal shoulders—adequate anaesthesia is necessary
  —if the above fail, try to deliver posterior shoulder and consider symphisiotomy.

MULTIPLE PREGNANCY AND LABOUR
TWINS

- Pre-term labour is common
- Placenta praevia may be present
- Prolapse of the cord must be watched for
- Malpresentations are more likely—the presentations in order of frequency being:
  - —Vertex: vertex
  - —Vertex: breech
  - —Breech: vertex
  - —Breech: breech
  - —Vertex: transverse
  - —Breech: transverse.

POSSIBLE INDICATIONS FOR ELECTIVE CAESAREAN SECTION

- First twin presenting as a breech
- Pre-term labour (before 34 weeks)
- Triplets (?) and higher multiples
- Proteinuric pre-eclampsia
- Any indication which would also apply in singleton pregnancies, e.g. IUGR, APH.

MANAGEMENT OF LABOUR AND DELIVERY

- An intravenous line should be set up and an anaesthetist should be present for delivery lest rapid general anaesthesia becomes necessary.
- After vaginal delivery of the first twin the second sac should be ruptured once uterine activity begins.
- If contractions do not begin within 15 minutes commence an oxytocin infusion.
- If the cord of the second twin prolapses proceed to ventouse extraction (if the presentation is cephalic) or breech extraction (if the presentation is breech).
- Anaesthesia for the latter should be epidural if already established, or general.
- The interval between delivery of the first and second twin should be no more than 20 minutes.
- Beware of postpartum haemorrhage.
- After delivery check placentae and membranes for zygosity. Histological confirmation is necessary.

OPERATIVE OBSTETRICS
EPISIOTOMY

- The need for an episiotomy is a matter for experienced clinical judgment.
- It should never be carried out merely because 'it is routine'.

- Too many episiotomies are performed in modern obstetrics and there is little evidence that the number of vaginal lacerations is reduced.

Indications
Among these will be:
- when a perineal tear appears inevitable otherwise
- in cases of fetal distress late in the second stage
- most forceps deliveries (except low cavity forceps)
- pre-term delivery
- breech delivery
- failure to advance because of perineal rigidity.

Technique
An episiotomy must be:
- performed at the correct time—incise too early and unnecessary blood loss will result
- carried out with adequate local or regional anaesthesia. Failure to use anaesthesia is to be deprecated
- made with sharp scissors in the correct place. The medio-lateral episiotomy is more common in the UK but the risks of the midline incision have been exaggerated. The episiotomy must always start in the midline
- repaired properly within as short a time of delivery as possible.

Side-effects
- *Pain.* This can be severe and is the main reason for avoiding episiotomy. It can be reduced by prompt, careful and expert repair.
- *Bleeding.* The average blood loss is about 100 ml and much larger losses are all too common.
- *Breakdown.* Inversely related to the expertise of the person repairing the episiotomy.
  —Potential causes are delay in suturing, inappropriate suture materials, bad technique
  —Primary repair with antibiotic cover should be carried out where possible.
- *Dyspareunia.* This can be so severe that it becomes a factor in marital breakdown.

THIRD-DEGREE TEAR

- The vaginal laceration or episiotomy has extended to involve at least the anal mucosa.
- It must be repaired in theatre under epidural or general anaesthesia by an experienced obstetrician.
- Give a low-residue diet and a faeces-softening agent (e.g. Normacol) for 1 week followed by a high-bulk diet.
- If the repair breaks down, eradicate local sepsis before attempting another repair.

INSTRUMENTAL DELIVERY

- Delivery can be by the vacuum extractor (ventouse) or obstetric forceps.
- The ventouse must not be considered as an easy way out when adverse features are present or the position of the fetal head is unknown.

Potential indications

- Failure to advance in the second stage, frequently due to failure of maternal effort, epidural analgesia and/or malposition of the fetal head
- Maternal conditions in which (prolonged) expulsive efforts may be detrimental, e.g. cardiac and respiratory disease, severe pre-eclampsia or eclampsia
- 'Fetal distress' in the second stage
- Prolapse of the cord in the second stage.

Prior conditions for instrumental delivery

- A legitimate indication must be present.
- The presentation must be suitable, i.e. vertex, face (mento-anterior) or after-coming head in a breech delivery.
- There must be no cephalo-pelvic disproportion. Moulding of the fetal skull must not be excessive.
- The head must be engaged. Ideally no part of the fetal head should be palpable per abdomen, and if more than one fifth can be palpated, vaginal delivery must not be contemplated.
- The position of the head must be known.
- For forceps, the cervix must be fully dilated.
- The ventouse can be used before the cervix has reached full dilatation (see below).
- Analgesia must be adequate.
- The bladder must be empty.
- The uterus must be contracting.

Forceps to the after-coming head (ACH) in a breech delivery

This is the method of choice for delivery of the ACH because of the degree of control the operator can exercise.

Forceps in the delivery of low birthweight (LBW) infants (<2500 g)

Lift-out forceps neither protects against nor induces birth trauma in LBW infants. Their use is therefore optional. Rotational forceps are best avoided for LBW infants.

Trial of forceps

- This is justifiable when it is likely, but not entirely certain, that vaginal delivery by forceps will be successful.
- Otherwise the patient should be delivered by caesarean section.

- Trial should be carried out in a theatre fully prepared for caesarean section.

The use of the ventouse
Vaginal delivery is said to be feasible from 5 cm. The following points are a guide to proper use of the ventouse:
- the patient's expulsive efforts are used to assist delivery
- the fetal head must be at least at the level of the spines
- the largest possible of the four cups should be used
- if delivery is not imminent after pulling on the ventouse during three contractions the attempt must cease and the patient must be delivered by caesarean section.

Analgesia for instrumental delivery
- Perineal infiltration alone is suitable for episiotomy, and low outlet deliveries using the ventouse or 'outlet' forceps.
- Pudendal nerve block is useful for mid-cavity forceps and some ventouse deliveries. It does not provide adequate analgesia for rotational forceps. The transvaginal route is recommended for insertion of the block.
- Epidural anaesthesia is ideal particularly for rotational forceps; it is also suitable for emergency caesarean sections in which an existing epidural block is providing good analgesia.

CAESAREAN SECTION

- In 1994–95 the overall caesarean rate in the UK was about 10.5% and has been rising since then. There are wide variations between regions and individual hospitals.
- *It must not be carried out without good reasons.*
- It is indicated when delivery must be effected rapidly for fetal and/or maternal reasons and when it is not thought to be safe vaginally.
- The transperitoneal lower segment caesarean section (LSCS) accounts for virtually all of the operations in modern obstetrics.
- Classical caesarean section is very occasionally indicated, e.g. for transverse lie with PROM, or for caesarean section at 26–28 weeks. In this latter situation the vertical incision starts in the lower segment but extends into the upper segment.

EPIDURAL OR SPINAL ANAESTHESIA AND CAESAREAN SECTION

Advantages
- The mother is awake and sees the child at delivery.
- The father can usually be present.
- Consciousness is not impaired immediately postoperatively. Postoperative problems and pain are less than after general anaesthesia.

- Breast-feeding and mobilisation can start early.

Disadvantages
- The procedure takes longer.
- Sometimes anaesthesia is not complete. Therefore the patient should be fully prepared for general anaesthesia (GA).
- Contraindications to epidural/spinal anaesthesia are discussed on page 137.

SOME IMPORTANT TECHNICAL POINTS ABOUT LSCS (LOWER SEGMENT CAESAREAN SECTION)

- H_2-receptor antagonists should be given pre-operatively to reduce the risk from aspiration of acid gastric contents.
- This also applies to procedures using epidural/spinal block lest conversion to GA becomes necessary.
- Induction of GA should take place at the last possible moment to reduce fetal exposure to the anaesthetic agents.
- The operation is carried out with a $10–15^0$ left lateral tilt to prevent supine hypotension.
- A cuffed endotracheal tube must be used.
- Special care must be taken in Rh-negative women to remove residual blood from the peritoneal cavity because some of it may be Rh-D-positive fetal blood.
- Thrombo-prophylaxis must be considered (see p. 102). At least early ambulation should be encouraged to reduce the risk of thromboembolism.

DELIVERY IN SUBSEQUENT PREGNANCIES

- Elective caesarean section is advised if the cause is recurrent (e.g. CPD).
- If vaginal delivery is attempted, oxytocin must be used only with the strongest of indications. (It may be helpful to monitor intrauterine pressure.)
- Epidural anaesthesia can be used; the pain of ruptured uterus will break through the epidural block.

MATERNAL MORTALITY AND CAESAREAN SECTION

- There were 98 direct and indirect maternal deaths due to caesarean section in the UK in 1991–93.
- There was a fall of 44% in deaths associated with elective caesarean sections compared with the previous triennium (17% v. 36%).
- A similar percentage *rise* in deaths occurred among 'unplanned emergency procedures' (19 v. 9 deaths). There was also an increase in the number after 'planned emergency' procedures (63% v. 52%) often because inexperienced junior staff took or were given too much responsibility.

- Substandard care was deemed to be a factor in 34%, the main criticisms being:
  —lack of facilities and staff for 'high risk' cases
  —failure to understand the severity of the woman's condition
  —misjudgment of fluid balance and transfusion requirements
  —inappropriate deputising or assumption of responsibility.
- The main associated causes of death (in order) were:
  —pulmonary embolism   14%
  —haemorrhage   11%
  —hypertensive complications   8%
  —sepsis   8%
  —anaesthetic complications   7%
  —other direct causes   16%
  —(indirect and fortuitous   36%)
- Of the nine *perimortem* caesarean sections, 9 from 11 babies survived; no babies survived from the 5 *postmortem* operations. Clear guidelines should be set for these procedures and made known in all Obstetric and Accident & Emergency Units. (*Perimortem* = mother close to death, unconscious, on CPR support and failed to regain consciousness after delivery.)

FURTHER READING

Birde R, Brooke L A, Gardosi J, Gibb D, Macdonald S E, Stirk F D, Weindling M A 1995 Clinical focus: shoulder dystocia. Clinical Risk 1:49–73

Chalmers I, Enkin M, Keirse M J N C 1989 Effective care in pregnancy and childbirth, Vol 2: Childbirth. Oxford University Press, Oxford

Chamberlain G (ed) 1995 Turnbull's Obstetrics. Churchill Livingstone, Edinburgh

The Cochrane Collaboration 1995 Cochrane Pregnancy and Childbirth Database. BMJ Publications, London

Creasy R K, Resnik R (eds) 1994 Maternal–fetal medicine—principles and practice. Saunders, Philadelphia

Greene K R 1987 The CG waveform. Clinical Obstetrics and Gynaecology 1:131–155

Hibbard B M, Anderson M A, Drife J O, Tighe J R et al 1996 Report on confidential enquiries into maternal deaths in the United Kingdom 1991–3 (and continuing triennial series). HMSO, London

Iams J D et al 1996 The length of the cervix and the risk of spontaneous premature delivery. New England Journal of Medicine 334:567–572

James D K, Steer P J, Weiner C P, Gonik B 1994 High risk pregnancy—management options. Saunders, London

McLean M, Walters A W A, Smith R 1993 Prediction and early diagnosis of preterm labour: a critical review. Obstetrical and Gynaecological Survey 48:209–225

O'Driscoll K, Meagher D, Boylan P 1993 Active management of labour, 3rd edn. Mosby-Wolfe, London

Rice G E, Brennecke S P 1993 Preterm labour and delivery. Clinical Obstetrics and Gynaecology 7:477–671

Rosevear S K, Stirrat G M 1996 Handbook of obstetric managment. Blackwell Scientific, Oxford

11. Third-stage problems and obstetric emergencies

THE NORMAL THIRD STAGE OF LABOUR

This beings with delivery of the baby and ends with expulsion of the placenta.

Management

'Physiological' management of the third stage involves:
- division of the umbilical cord only when pulsation has ceased
- delivery of the placenta by maternal effort and aided by gravity without cord traction
- use of oxytocics only if haemorrhage occurs.

This policy allows blood volume to equilibrate between mother and baby and avoids side-effects of oxytocin.

'Active' management of the third stage has become routine over the past 20 years in the UK and is associated with reduced blood loss overall. This involves:
- syntometrine (syntocinon 5 units: ergometrine 0.5 mg) with delivery of the anterior shoulder
- delivery of the placenta by *controlled cord traction (CCT)* when separation has occurred.

POSTPARTUM HAEMORRHAGE (PPH) AND RETAINED PLACENTA

Definition
Primary postpartum haemorrhage is the loss of 500 ml or more of blood within 24 hours of delivery.

Incidence
- Incidence varies from 2 to 8% among hospitals.
- It accounted for eight maternal deaths in the UK in 1991–93: four of these women were aged 30 or over.

Associated factors
These are listed in the information box.

Postpartum haemorrhage and retained placenta: associated factors

- High multiparity (associated with uterine atony)
- Maternal age 35 or over
- Delivery after an APH
- Multiple pregnancy
- Polyhydramnios
- Past history of PPH (due to placenta praevia or abruptio placentae)
- Coagulation disorders

Main causes
- Retained placenta (in part or whole)
- Uterine atony
- Soft tissue lacerations.

Management
Prevention Proper management of the third stage, e.g. do not 'fiddle' with the uterine fundus while waiting for placental separation.

Treatment
- Rub up a uterine contraction.
- Correct hypovolaemia by intravenous fluids and screened Group O, Rh-D negative, Kell-negative blood if necessary.
- Remove the placenta if it is retained or incomplete using general or epidural anaesthesia.
- Check for vaginal, cervical or uterine lacerations.
- Maintain uterine contraction with an oxytocin infusion.
- Deal with coagulation failure as described on page 163.

Management of massive haemorrhage
(see Hibbard et al in Further Reading)
- **Prompt and decisive action is necessary: every labour ward must have a protocol for management with which all staff are familiar.**
- Summon all extra staff required—obstetricians, anaesthetists, midwives, porters (to relay samples and fetch blood).
- Alert haematologist and blood transfusion service.
- Set up at least two large infusion lines.
- Monitor CVP, intra-arterial pressure, heart rate, ECG, PO_2 and urine output.
- Send at least 20 ml of blood for cross-matching and coagulation screen. **Order a minimum of 6 units of blood**.
- Give warmed whole blood if possible (under pressure if necessary); but if only plasma reduced blood is available, infuse additional colloid if more than 3 units are given.

- Do not give FFP or platelets until haemorrhage has stopped or at least 5 units of stored blood have been given. Avoid dextran. **The primary aim is to restore circulating volume**.
- Internal iliac ligation and/or hysterectomy are rarely necessary. If indicated, laparotomy must be embarked on before the situation is desperate.

MORBID ADHERENCE OF THE PLACENTA (PLACENTA ACCRETA)

- This is a rare occurrence. As much of the placenta as possible should be removed manually under GA and the uterus packed. Transfusion will be necessary.
- Severe degrees of placenta accreta will require hysterectomy.

CORD PRESENTATION AND PROLAPSE

- Cord presentation discovered before rupture of the membranes is an indication for immediate caesarean section.
- Cord prolapse is associated with all factors maintaining the presenting part high above the pelvis or when it does not fit well into the pelvis at the time of rupture of the membranes, e.g:
  —transverse lie —pre-term labour
  —polyhydramnios —multiple pregnancy
  —CPD —breech presentation.

Diagnosis
The cord is visible or palpable. Consider if fetal distress occurs in association with spontaneous rupture of the membranes.

Management
Management depends on whether or not the child is alive.
- If it is, and the cervix is fully dilated, expedite delivery with forceps (or breech extraction perhaps).
- If the cervix is not fully dilated, arrange urgent caesarean section.

EMERGENCY PROCEDURES

- Displace the presenting part with the examining hand.
- Fill the bladder with 750 ml of normal saline by indwelling catheter.
- Drop the end of the bed or stretcher.
- Keep the patient in the knee–elbow position until delivery can be effected.

UTERINE RUPTURE

Uterine rupture caused three maternal deaths in the UK from 1991–93. The main associated factors are:
- previous caesarean section scar (often classical)

- the inappropriate use of oxytocin to augment labour (e.g. in multiparous women)
- previous cervical surgery
- failure to recognise obstructed labour.

Signs and symptoms
- Anything from lower abdominal discomfort to severe 'bursting' pain (which will even break through an epidural block)
- Unexplained maternal tachycardia
- Variable amounts of vaginal bleeding
- Fainting and ensuing shock
- Cessation of contractions
- Disappearance of the presenting part from the pelvis
- Fetal distress
- Possibility of an unrecognised rupture must be considered when bleeding continues after delivery despite well-retracted uterus, or there is unexplained shock (particularly if mother was delivered by forceps or has had a previous caesarean section).

Management
- Arrange immediate laparotomy
- Replace circulating volume—as for major haemorrhage
- Carry out the least extensive surgery compatible with the patient's immediate health and future welfare
- Take great care to identify the ureters and exclude them from any sutures.

Future pregnancies
Close observation is required during any future pregnancy, and delivery should be by elective caesarean section at 38 weeks.

UTERINE INVERSION

- This is a profoundly shocking complication.
- It is often caused by injudicious cord traction with an atonic uterus when the insertion of the placenta is fundal.
- The inversion may not be complete and therefore not immediately visible. Diagnosis is by vaginal examination.

Management
- Try to reduce the inversion.
- Initiate anti-shock measures.
- If the placenta is still attached and easy to remove, do so, once the shock has been corrected.
- The hydrostatic method for reduction is usually effective:
  —the inverted uterus is held within the vagina
  —2 litres of warm saline are infused rapidly into the vagina and the even hydrostatic pressure exerted usually reduces the inverted uterus.

AMNIOTIC FLUID EMBOLISM

This caused 10 maternal deaths in the UK in 1991–93.

Associated factors
- Precipitate labour
- Polyhydramnios
- Hypertonic uterine action (with or without oxytocin)
- Induction or augmentation of labour with prostaglandin pessaries.

Signs and symptoms
- Profound shock
- Cyanosis
- Dyspnoea leading to respiratory arrest
- Severe coagulation defect.

Management
- Prevent death from pulmonary vascular obstruction by endotracheal intubation and administration of oxygen and hydrocortisone (i.v.)
- Control coagulation defect.

COAGULATION FAILURE

Main causes in pregnancy
- Placental abruption
- Amniotic fluid embolism
- Endotoxic shock.

Diagnosis
- Clinical observation
- Whole blood clotting time (normal 5–10 minutes)
- Thrombin clotting time—a sample of blood added to a tube containing a small amount of thrombin should clot within 10 seconds
- Reduction in platelet count
- Reduced fibrinogen titres
- Increased levels of fibrin degradation products.

Management
- The coagulation defect is usually self-limiting if the stimulus producing it is removed. Therefore the uterus should be emptied as expeditiously as possible.
- Transfuse—see Management of massive haemorrhage (p. 160).

ACUTE ABDOMINAL PAIN IN PREGNANCY

The differential diagnosis of acute abdominal pain can be difficult in pregnancy.

CAUSES INCIDENTAL TO PREGNANCY

Examples include:
- appendicitis (see below)
- accident to ovarian cyst
- acute cholecystitis
- renal calculus
- intestinal obstruction
- volvulus
- perforated peptic ulcer
- rectus abdominis haematoma.

CAUSES RELATED TO PREGNANCY

Causes may be related to early or later pregnancy, as indicated in the information box.

Early pregnancy	Later pregnancy
• Abortion (including septic)	• Abruptio placentae
• Cornual pregnancy (or other ectopic pregnancy)	• Uterine rupture
• Acute retention of urine	• Severe pre-eclampsia
• Due to retroverted gravid uterus	• Degeneration of fibroid
	• Pyelonephritis
	• Extrauterine pregnancy

Appendicitis can be difficult to diagnose in pregnancy because:
- the appendix is displaced upward
- the site of pain is often atypical
- examination is made difficult by the pregnant uterus
- the body's reaction (e.g. leucocytosis) may be masked.

FURTHER READING

Chamberlain G (ed) 1995 Turnbull's obstetrics. Churchill Livingstone, Edinburgh

Creasy R K Resnik R (eds) 1994 Maternal–fetal medicine—principles and practice, 3rd edn. Saunders, Philadelphia

Enkin M, Keirse M J N C, Chalmers I 1989 Effective care in pregnancy and childbirth, Vol. 2: Childbirth. Oxford University Press, Oxford

Hibbard B M, Anderson M A, Drife J O, Tighe J R et al 1996 Report on confidential enquiries into maternal deaths in the United Kingdom 1991–1993 (and continuing triennial series). HMSO, London

Rosevear S K, Stirrat G M 1996 Handbook of obstetric management. Blackwell Scientific, Oxford

12. Perinatal and maternal mortality

DEFINITIONS

Livebirth The complete expulsion or extraction from its mother of a product of conception, irrespective of gestational age, which then breathes or shows any evidence of life such as beating of the heart, pulsation of the umbilical cord, or definite movement of voluntary muscles.

Stillbirth Birth of an infant who shows no evidence of life after birth.

Death, fetal (prenatal death) Death of a fetus in utero which, at birth, weighs 500 g or more irrespective of gestational age.

Death, infant, early neonatal Death of a liveborn infant occurring less than 7 completed days (168 hours) from the time of birth.

Death, infant, late neonatal Death of a liveborn infant after 7 completed days of age but before 28 completed days.

The perinatal period
- Commences when a fetus has developed to a weight of 1000 g (approximately equivalent to 28 weeks' gestation); ends when the newborn baby has achieved an age of 7 completed days (168 hours) of life.
- In the absence of measured birthweight, a body length of 35 cm is considered equivalent to 1000 g birthweight.
- When neither birthweight nor body length has been measured, a fetus is considered to have entered the perinatal period when the gestational age has reached 28 completed weeks (196 days).

PERINATAL MORTALITY

- The perinatal mortality rate (PMR) is now the number of stillbirths and first-week deaths occurring from 24 (previously 28) completed weeks of pregnancy to 7 days after birth per 1000 live and stillbirths.
- If an infant is born before 24 weeks' gestation and shows signs of life but then dies within 7 days it is included as a perinatal death.
- The RCOG recommends that births from 20 weeks' gestation (or fetal weight 300 g and above if gestation not known) should be notified.

- National perinatal statistics should include, as minima, infants with birthweight >500 g *or* at least 22 completed weeks or crown–heel length at least 25 cm.
- For international statistics the minima should be birthweight 1000 g, gestational age 28 weeks *or* crown–heel length 35 cm.
- In 1994 the mortality rates in England and Wales were as follows:
  —perinatal mortality rate: 8.9/1000 live and stillbirths
  —infant mortality rate: 6.2/1000 livebirths (the lowest rate ever recorded)
  —neonatal mortality rate: 4.1/1000 livebirths.

IMMEDIATE CAUSES OF PERINATAL DEATH

The main determinants are:
- low (<2500 g) and very low <1500 g) birthweight about 30% of total
- congenital anomalies about 20%
- antepartum haemorrhage about 15%
- maternal disorder about 10%
- pre-eclampsia about 5%
- (unexplained over 2500 g about 10%).

FACTORS INFLUENCING PMR

Birthweight
- PMR and birthweight are closely related. The lowest rate occurs over 3000 g.
- 60% of perinatal deaths occurred in the 6.5% of babies born weighing <2500 g.
- 36% of perinatal deaths occurred in the 1% of babies <1500 g.
- IUGR is associated with a four-fold increase in PMR even when the association with congenital anomalies is excluded.

Social class
- Perinatal mortality rises as social class falls.
- This is partly explained by smoking.

Maternal age and parity
- The PMR is at its lowest in mothers between the ages of 25 and 29 years and for the second child.
- It increases three-fold for mothers aged 40–44, doubles for the fifth child, and trebles for the seventh.
- This is influenced by social class and the association of congenital anomalies with age.

Race
- The PMR is raised among immigrants from Pakistan, East and West Africa and the West Indies.

Multiple births
See page 125.

PERINATAL MORTALITY RATES

- Perinatal mortality (PNM) rates are commonly used as an indicator of standards of obstetric care.
- This is inappropriate for the following reasons:
  —international comparisons are confounded by different definitions
  —in the developed world perinatal death is no longer common enough to allow it to be used in this way. In the developing world data collection is incomplete
  —60% of the deaths remain unexplained and are not associated with any risk marker
  —two of the major contributors, lethal congenital malformations and very pre-term delivery, cannot truly be prevented by obstetric care
  —up to 25% of the decline in PNM can be explained by increases in birthweight due to socioeconomic changes
  —much of the remaining decline is due to improvements in neonatal rather than obstetric care.

PERINATAL MORBIDITY

- There are no national statistics available for perinatal morbidity or subsequent disability; neither is there any agreed definition of disability.
- It is not at all clear that the incidence of disability will fall as mortality is reduced.
- It is also still not clear what factors affect the developmental achievements of children and why one child suffers while another does not.

THE MANAGEMENT OF INTRAUTERINE FETAL DEATH (IUFD)

- If an IUFD is suspected, confirm by ultrasound scan.
- No fetal heart or movement can be detected and there may be overlap of skull bones in the absence of labour.
- If confirmed, discuss with the parents possible explanation, plans for management and the future.
- *Sensitive and sympathetic support for the mother and family are vital at all times.*
- Labour can be induced with vaginal prostaglandins (see p. 135).

PERINATAL PATHOLOGY

Good regional perinatal pathology services are fundamental to the practice of high-standard obstetrics and neonatal medicine.

PROCEDURES IN THE EVENT OF A PERINATAL DEATH

- *Detailed inspection and measurement of the baby.* The minimum requirements are:
  —measure weight, crown–heel, crown–rump, and foot lengths and occipito-frontal circumference
  —look for malformations, deformations, state of maceration (if any) and evidence of trauma. Pay special attention to limbs, genitalia and facies.
- *Detailed clinical information* must be supplied to the pathologist (preferably on a structured request form), who should also have access to the casenotes.
- *Request an autopsy* in all cases, even when the cause seems obvious:
  —it is the right of each couple to have as much information as possible
  —autopsy rates of less than 75% suggest a poor perinatal service
  —in the case of stillbirth, submit fetus and placenta together
  —the placenta of every baby born weighing less than 1500 g and/or less than the third percentile for gestational age and sex, and of all multiple pregnancies, should be sent for examination because these babies are at greatest risk of neonatal death.
- *Maternal investigations* are the responsibility of the obstetrician. These should include (as a minimum): TORCH screen, Kleihauer test, VDRL and Rh or other antibodies if not checked antenatally, random blood sugar and glycosylated Hb or fructosamine.
- *The extent of the further investigation* of the baby depends on the autopsy findings, measurements and histological examination (of baby and placenta). These are the guide to further cytogenetic, biochemical, microbiological or haematological investigations required. If dwarfism is suspected, X-ray examination is mandatory.
- The parents must be treated with the utmost compassion and be encouraged (but not forced) to see their dead child even if disfiguring abnormalities are present.
  —A polaroid photograph should be taken and kept for the parents to see and keep when they wish
  —Informed assistance should be given with registration and funeral arrangements.
- The GP and community midwife must be informed quickly.
- The couple should be seen by the obstetrician (and paediatrician in the case of a neonatal death) when all the information on the case is available.

MATERNAL MORTALITY

DEFINITION

Maternal death The death of a woman while pregnant or within 42 days of delivery or abortion from any cause related to or aggravated by the pregnancy or its management (excluding accidental or incidental causes).

Direct death That resulting from obstetric complications of pregnancy, labour or the puerperium; from interventions, omissions, incorrect treatment, or from a chain of events resulting from any of these.

Indirect death That resulting from pre-existing disease, or a condition arising during pregnancy not due to direct obstetric causes but aggravated by the physiological changes in pregnancy.

Late death That occurring between 42 days and 1 year after abortion or delivery due to *direct* or *indirect* causes.

Fortuitous death That due to causes unrelated to, but occurring in, pregnancy, labour or the puerperium.

Substandard care Means that the care received (or made available to) the woman was deemed to fall below the 'contemporary standards of good practice'.

Maternal mortality rate Expressed per million 'maternities', i.e. pregnancy, childbirth or abortion.

Table 12.1 Main direct causes of maternal deaths in England and Wales 1985–1993 (rate per million maternities and [% of total deaths*]). Source: Hibbard et al 1996 (see Further Reading)

	1985–87	1988–90	1991–93
Pulmonary embolism	12.8 [23]	10.2 [23]	13 [27]
Hypertensive disorders	11.9 [19]	11.4 [19]	8.6 [15.5]
Anaesthesia	2.6 [4]	1.7 [3]	3.5 [6]
Amniotic fluid embolism	4.0 [6.5]	4.7 [8]	4.3 [7]
Abortion/ectopic pregnancy	2.6/7.1 [16]	3.8/6.4 [17]	3.5/3.5 [14]
Antepartum and postpartum haemorrhage	4.4 [7]	9.3 [15]	6.5 [12]
Genital tract sepsis	2.6 [4]	3.0 [5]	3.9 [7]
Genital tract trauma	2.6 [4]	1.3 [2]	1.7 [3]
Other direct deaths	9.2 [15]	5.9 [10]	4.3 [8]
Total [100%]	61.2	61.4	55.7

* to nearest whole number

- Each of the main causes is discussed in the relevant chapter.
- 'Substandard care' was thought to have contributed to the outcome in 40% of deaths in 1991–93:
  —30% related to hospital care; 7% to GP care; and 11% to the actions of the woman or her relatives

—it was a factor in 16 (85%) of hypertensive deaths, 11 (70%) deaths from haemorrhage, and all eight anaesthetic deaths.

FURTHER READING

Chamberlain G (ed) 1995 Turnbull's obstetrics. Churchill Livingstone, Edinburgh
Hibbard B M, Anderson M A, Drife J O, Tighe J R et al 1996 Report on confidential enquiries into maternal deaths in the United Kingdom 1991–93 (and continuing triennial series). HMSO, London
Rosevear S K, Stirrat G M 1996 Handbook of obstetric management. Blackwell Scientific, Oxford

13. The puerperium

- The puerperium is the period of time over which the genital tract returns to normal after childbirth.
- It is assumed to last 6 weeks.

THE NORMAL PUERPERIUM

Characterised by:
- lactation
- lochia
- involution of the uterus
- return of the genital tract to normal.

Breast-feeding
- Breast milk is every baby's birthright and every encouragement should be given to a woman to breast-feed. To do this:
  —inform all pregnant women about the technique and benefits of breast-feeding
  —give new mothers encouragement and assistance as they begin
  —give the baby no other food or drink than breast milk.
- Among the benefits are:
  —passive immunity from immunoglobulins in breast milk
  —fewer gastrointestinal symptoms
  —fewer neonatal seizures
  —lower incidence of auto-immune conditions (e.g. juvenile onset diabetes)
  —reduced risk of sudden infant death syndrome
  —psychological advantages for the baby
  —higher IQ(?)
- Breast-feeding is an effective contraceptive as long as the baby is having at least 5 feeds/24 hours.

Suppression of lactation
- This is seldom necessary now except, perhaps, after a perinatal death.
- Bromocriptine can be used.

Management of breast engorgement
- Firm support of breast with a good bra
- Adequate analgesia

- Warm bathing of breasts
- Expression should be avoided
- If needs be, bromocriptine can be prescribed.

PUERPERAL PYREXIA

- This is defined as a temperature of 38°C on any occasion in the first 14 days after delivery or miscarriage.
- A slight fever is not uncommon within the first 24 hours after delivery.
- Among the possible causes are:
  —urinary tract infection   —deep vein thrombosis
  —genital tract infection   —respiratory infection
  —breast infection   —other non-obstetric causes.
- Carry out a full clinical investigation (including breasts and legs) as well as an MSU, cervical and high vaginal swabs, blood culture and sputum culture (if possible).
- After the investigations have been sent to the laboratory, and if the clinical situation warrants it, antibiotic therapy can be started.

Mastitis

- *Acute intramammary mastitis* is due to failure of milk withdrawal from a lobule. Treatment involves getting the baby to empty the breast, cold compresses, and antibiotics if there is no improvement within 24 hours.
- *Infective mastitis* may be due to *Staph. aureus*, and treatment with an antibiotic to which that organism is sensitive may be necessary.
- *Breast abscess* formation is rare but preventable. Antibiotics are of value only if given early. An established abscess requires surgical drainage.

SECONDARY POSTPARTUM HAEMORRHAGE

- This is defined as excessive (amount is not specified) blood loss from the genital tract more than 24 hours after and within 6 weeks of delivery.
- Among the commonest causes are retained placental fragments or blood clot (usually within a few days of delivery) or infection (often later).
- If the bleeding has been slight and there is no evidence of infection the patient needs no more than to be kept under observation.
- Careful evacuation of the uterus under general anaesthesia is indicated if:
  —an ultrasound scan suggests the presence of retained products
  —heavy bleeding persists

—the uterus is larger than expected and tender; the cervix is
  open.
- Infection is treated appropriately.

PERINEAL PAIN

Prevention
Avoidance of trauma at delivery, and proper repair of tears or
episiotomy.

Treatment
- Local anaesthetic sprays relieve pain in the immediate
  postpartum period. There is no evidence that ice, salt or other
  baths, or herbal remedies, produce lasting benefit. Local steroids
  should be avoided.
- Relief of pressure on perineum.
- Ultrasound or pulsed electromagnetic energy—controlled trials
  show no clear benefit.
- Analgesia—paracetamol or NSAIDs for mild pain; unfortunately
  no analgesic seems to be of real value for severe pain.

EFFECTS OF CHILDBIRTH ON PELVIC FLOOR MUSCLES AND NERVES

- The pelvic floor muscles and nerves are damaged even by a
  normal delivery.
- Ventouse extraction is usually less traumatic than forceps.
- Obstetric trauma predisposes to faecal incontinence.
- Division of the external anal sphincter at delivery is associated
  with long-term and sometimes severe effects on anal canal
  sensation and function.

FURTHER READING

Chamberlain G (ed) 1995 Turnbull's obstetrics. Churchill Livingstone, Edinburgh
Rosevear S K, Stirrat G M 1996 Handbook of obstetric management. Blackwell
  Scientific, Oxford

14. The newborn infant

ASSESSMENT AT BIRTH

APGAR SCORE

This should be carried out on all babies at 1 and 5 minutes after birth.

Scores of 0 to 2 are given for each of the following parameters:
- heart rate
- respiratory effort
- muscle tone
- response to catheter in nostril
- colour.

A score of 7 or less at 5 minutes suggests some degree of 'birth asphyxia'.

Routine examination within 2 hours of birth

The object of the examination is to ask:
- is the baby pre-term or small-for-dates?
- is cyanosis, jaundice or anaemia apparent?
- is there evidence of birth trauma?
- are there any congenital anomalies (e.g. congenital dislocation of hips)?

ASSESSMENT OF GESTATIONAL AGE

- Gestational age can be assessed independently of knowledge of menstrual age using a score from a series of physical criteria (the Farr Score) which can be used alone or in combination with an assessment of neurological criteria (Dubowicz score).
- The total score can be translated into an estimate of gestational age. For further information see Further Reading.

RESUSCITATION

- The priorities of resuscitation are:
  —maintenance of body temperature
  —clearance of airways
  —establishment of ventilation (with or without administration of oxygen).

- Each obstetric unit should have:
  —all staff trained in basic bag and mask resuscitation
  —staff available trained in advanced resuscitation
  —regular training sessions in immediate neonatal care and resuscitation.
- More than 80% of babies will respond to resuscitation with bag and mask.
- Clear guidelines should be established for the extremely immature baby (<1000 g) and, if at all possible, discussed with the parents before delivery:
  —a clear prospective decision should be made (if possible) about resuscitation at <25 weeks
  —an experienced neonatal paediatrician needs to be present.
- The outcome for babies born with an Apgar score of zero *known to have been alive shortly before birth* is more encouraging than one would think. Of such babies:
  —50% survive intact, 25% die and 25% survive with significant disabilities
  —it is, therefore, suggested that active attempts should be made to establish circulation and resuscitate these babies.

INDICATIONS FOR THE PRESENCE OF NEONATAL PAEDIATRICIAN (OR EQUIVALENT) AT DELIVERY

- All caesarean sections
- All instrumental deliveries
- Pre-term delivery
- IUGR
- APH
- Polyhydramnios
- Multiple pregnancy
- Maternal history of diabetes
- ITP, myasthenia, thyrotoxicosis, drug abuse
- Fetal anomaly
- Suspected amnionitis
- Breech delivery
- Meconium staining of liquor
- Severe Rhesus (or other) iso-immunisation

ADMISSION TO SPECIAL CARE BABY UNIT (SCBU)

- Babies should not be separated from their mothers without good cause.
- The following babies usually need further special care on SCBU or transitional care ward:
  —after prolonged resuscitation
  —birthweight less than 2000 g
  —gestational age less than 36 weeks
  —persisting respiratory problem
  —some severe congenital anomalies
  —all ill babies
  —infants of drug-abusing mothers.
- The mother and father should be given an opportunity to see and hold the baby before transfer if at all possible.

NEONATAL SCREENING AND TREATMENT

PHENYLKETONURIA (PKU)

- The incidence is 1/10 000 livebirths.
- The Guthrie test or a chromatographic test should be carried out routinely within 7–14 days of delivery. If the Guthrie bacteriological test is used it should be postponed if the baby is on antibiotics.

CONGENITAL HYPOTHYROIDISM

- The incidence is about 1/4000 livebirths.
- Without a screening programme for its detection only 40% of cases will be diagnosed by 3 months of age.
- Hypothyroidism can lead to mental retardation unless treated early.
- Testing (on a dried blood filter-paper spot) can be carried out at the same time as for PKU. TSH alone or T_4 and TSH are measured.

CONGENITAL DISLOCATION OF THE HIP

If the hips are or can be dislocated, treat in an abduction splint (for 8–12 weeks) and refer to a paediatrician or orthopaedic surgeon.

BCG VACCINATION

BCG should be given:
- to newborn children in families known to have had tuberculosis whatever the type and however long ago
- to children of *all* Asian immigrant families (tuberculosis is still widespread in the Asian communities amongst people who have been in the country for some years)
- if the mother's sputum is positive for tuberculosis the baby should be given isoniazid-resistant BCG and treated with isoniazid. Baby and mother should be kept separate until the mother has been on anti-tuberculous treatment for 2 weeks.

OPHTHALMIA NEONATORUM

- This is defined as any purulent discharge from the eyes of an infant starting within 21 days of birth.
- It is still a notifiable disease and can cause severe damage if not treated promptly and adequately. Among the causes are:
  —*Neisseria gonorrhoeae*
  —Other bacteria
  —*Chlamydia trachomatis.*
- Treatment should be in consultation with an ophthalmologist and venereologist.

NEONATAL JAUNDICE

- If a term baby becomes jaundiced, note date of onset, method of feeding, maternal blood group, history of perinatal trauma, and use of large volume of syntocinon-containing fluid during labour.
- Investigate bilirubin level >200 μmol/L within 48 hours of birth. Check:
  —proportion of direct bilirubin in blood
  —blood group of mother and baby
  —Coombs' test and other antibodies
  —FBC, reticulocytes and differential white cell count
  —urine for microscopy and reducing substances
  —thyroid function tests
  —glucose-6-phosphate dehydrogenase assay.
- Phototherapy will reduce the level and extent of the jaundice. It disrupts contact between baby and parents, who may find it distressing. It is of no proven value for term infants over 48 hours of age with bilirubin levels <300 μmol/L.

DISCHARGE EXAMINATION

- All babies should be examined in the presence of the mother before going home in order to:
  —assess his or her progress from birth
  —exclude malformations or traumatic lesions missed earlier
  —identify any superficial infections
  —reassure the mother.
- The following should be checked:
  —baby's general appearance
  —superficial infections (and other lesions) of eyes, mouth, umbilicus, nails
  —heart for murmurs
  —abdomen (**NB** The liver is normally 1–2 cm palpable)
  —male genitalia for hypospadias, undescended testes, herniae and hydroceles
  —female genitalia for vaginal discharge, fused labia, enlarged clitoris
  —hips for congenital dislocation ⎫ Discuss with orthopaedic
  —feet for talipes equino varus ⎭ surgeon if present.

FURTHER READING

Fleming P J, Speidel B D, Dunn P M 1991 A neonatal vade mecum, 2nd edn. Arnold, London

15. Obstetrics in developing countries

- Childbirth is still the main cause of death of females of reproductive age in developing countries.
- Probably more than 90% of pregnant women throughout the world deliver without ever having been in contact with anyone formally trained in any form of obstetric care.
- Antenatal, intrapartum and postpartum care is supervised by the traditional birth attendant, all too often in the context of malnutrition, infection and unregulated fertility.
- Even uncontaminated water is unavailable for the majority of the world's pregnant women.
- Even when lack of care is not due to ignorance, bad communication and lack of transport make contact with a clinic or hospital impossible, particularly during heavy rains or other severe climatic conditions.
- The following are among the particular problems which affect even those fortunate enough to have access to the most basic care:
  —illegal abortion
  —trophoblastic tumours (particularly Latin America, Far East and Eastern Asia)
  —severe anaemia
  —malaria
  —HIV, hepatitis and other infections (particularly STDs)
  —pre-eclampsia and eclampsia
  —antepartum and postpartum haemorrhage
  —obstructed labour (resulting in rupture of the uterus, stillbirth and/or obstetric fistulae)
  —sepsis.
- The incidence of low birthweight is high, due both to pre-term labour and IUGR.

MATERNAL MORTALITY IN DEVELOPING COUNTRIES

- WHO reports overall maternal mortality rates (MMR) in developing countries of between 1 and 4/1000 births rising to 78/1000 among unbooked patients in Indonesia (cf. UK <0.1/1000 births).
- The main causes overall are abortion, anaemia, eclampsia, haemorrhage, sepsis, and obstructed labour and its consequences.

PERINATAL MORTALITY IN DEVELOPING COUNTRIES

- Perinatal mortality rates (PMR) are said to range from 35 to 80/1000 births, but in most developing countries the true picture is unknown.
- Infection is the main perinatal hazard, particularly in low-birthweight babies.
- However, among the other main causes are intrapartum asphyxia, meconium aspiration, pre-eclampsia and syphilis.
- Traditional practices account for a high incidence of tetanus neonatorum.

REMEDIES

- Western-style medicine is inappropriate because its high-cost technology cannot be properly maintained and it takes finances away from more locally appropriate care.
- Socioeconomic remedies are paramount, with improved fertility control and greater status for women in society.
- A hospital-based programme of obstetric care is beyond reach of every developing country and is not appropriate for any but high-risk patients.
- Thus, when services are planned they must be practical (i.e. achievable now) and form a basis for future development and extension.
- The only possible basis for such care is specially trained midwives and nursing staff working in basic clinics accessible to the homes of the women.
  —An obstetrically trained doctor supervises them from the base hospital
  —Strict criteria for referral of patients to the base hospital must be laid down and adhered to
  —High-risk patients may require immediate transfer to the hospital; emergency transport is therefore absolutely vital.

SECTION TWO
Gynaecology

16. Disorders of menstruation and associated problems

AMENORRHOEA

Definitions
- *Primary amenorrhoea:*
—no menstruation by the age of 14 years accompanied by failure to grow properly or develop secondary sexual characteristics, *or*
—no menstruation by the age of 16 when growth and sexual development are normal.

- *Secondary amenorrhoea:* the absence of menses for 6 months (or greater than three times the previous cycle intervals) in a woman who has menstruated before.

When diagnoses are being considered, these 'primary' and 'secondary' categories must not be adhered to too rigidly.

Causes
If the amenorrhoea is not physiological (pre-pubertal, pregnancy, post-menopausal) it may be due to:
- disorders of outflow tract and/or uterus
- disorders of ovary
- disorders of hypothalamo-pituitary axis.

DISORDERS OF THE OUTFLOW TRACT AND/OR UTERUS

Cryptomenorrhoea
Vaginal atresia or an imperforate hymen prevents menstrual loss from escaping.

Features Primary amenorrhoea in a teenage girl with normal sexual development complaining of:
- intermittent abdominal pain
- possible difficulty with micturition
- palpable lower abdominal swelling
- bulging, bluish membrane at lower end of vagina.

Management Incise membrane under aseptic conditions.

Absence or hypoplasia of vagina
Features
- Growth, development and ovarian function are usually normal.

- The uterus is usually absent if only the lower third of the vagina has developed but may be normal or rudimentary.
- Renal anomalies (in 30%) or skeletal defects (in 10%) may be present also.

Management A functional vagina can be created by surgery or by dilators.

Testicular feminisation
The phenotype is female but the genotype is XY, and testes are present. It is inherited by an X-linked recessive gene resulting in absence of cytosol androgen receptors.

Features
- Growth and development are normal (may be taller than average and eunuchoid)
- Breasts are large but with sparse glandular tissue, nipples and pale areolae
- Inguinal herniae occur in 50% of cases (usually bilateral)
- Little or no axillary and pubic hair
- Labia minora are underdeveloped
- The vagina is blind ending, the uterus absent and the fallopian tubes rudimentary
- The testes are in the abdomen or inguinal canals
- Normal levels of testosterone are produced but there is no response to androgens (endogenous or exogenous)
- There is no spermatogenesis
- There is a high risk of testicular neoplasia (50%) if the testes are not removed shortly after puberty.

Consider the diagnosis in a female child:
- with bilateral inguinal herniae
- with primary amenorrhoea and absent uterus
- when body hair is absent.

Management
- These patients should be treated as female.
- The gonads should be removed after puberty and oestrogen replacement therapy started.
- Rare cases of incomplete testicular feminisation do occur. They have a variable degree of masculinisation.

Asherman's syndrome
Secondary amenorrhoea following destruction of the endometrium by overzealous curettage. Multiple synechiae show up on hysterography.

Management Break down intrauterine adhesions through a hysteroscope and insert an IUD for 10–12 months to deter reformation.

Infection

For example: tuberculosis and uterine schistosomiasis.

DISORDERS OF THE OVARY

Chromosomal abnormalities

Turner's syndrome (45X)—gonadal dysgenesis.

Features
- Amenorrhoea (primary but rarely secondary) ⎫
- Short stature   ⎬ most constant
- Failure of secondary sexual development   ⎭ features
- Webbing of the neck
- Increasing carrying angle ⎫
- Shield chest.   ⎬ less common
- Coarctation of aorta   ⎭
- Renal collecting system defects

Streak ovaries are present; gonadotrophins are high and oestrogens low. A mosaic chromosome pattern (e.g. XX/XO) will lead to various degrees of gonadal dysgenesis, secondary amenorrhoea and premature menopause.

Management
- Short stature may be treated if the diagnosis is made early, by use of oxandrolone and/or growth hormone before commencing oestrogen replacement therapy.
- If a Y chromosome is present in the genotype the risk of gonadal malignancy makes gonadectomy advisable.

Failure of gonadal development
- Gonadal agenesis—see page 246.

Resistant ovary syndrome
- A rare condition in which FSH is elevated despite normal ovarian development and potential.
- It may resolve spontaneously or intermittently. In rare cases ovulation may be induced by a combination of ethinyl oestradiol (to try to induce ovarian gonadotrophin receptors) and exogenous gonadotrophin therapy. Otherwise no treatment is possible except hormone replacement therapy (see p. 296).

Premature menopause
- See page 295.

DISORDERS OF THE HYPOTHALAMO-PITUITARY AXIS

Hyperprolactinaemia

- Prolactin is controlled primarily by inhibition by dopamine from the hypothalamus. It is not subject to negative feedback by peripheral hormones.
- Hyperprolactinaemia is defined as levels of >800 mU/L. It is only clinically significant if accompanied by oligomenorrhoea.
- It accounts for 20% of women with amenorrhoea and 2% with oligomenorrhoea. Hyperprolactinaemia interferes with the menstrual cycle by indirect suppression of the pulsatility of LH secretion.
- Women with prolonged hyperprolactinaemic amenorrhoea are at risk of osteoporosis.
- Galactorrhoea occurs in <50% of women with hyperprolactinaemia.
- Among the potential causes are:
  —'idiopathic' (about 40% of cases)—levels are usually <2500 mU/L. (Beware spurious diagnosis due to misinterpretation of results!)
  —prolactin-secreting 'tumours' (40–50%); most are 'microadenomas' (i.e <10 mm diameter)—it is arguable whether these are true neoplasms. A macroadenoma is to be expected if prolactin levels exceed 2500–3000 mU/L
  —other tumours compressing the pituitary stalk (rare—e.g. craniopharyngioma)
  —primary hypothyroidism (3–5%)
  —drugs (1–2%)—metoclopramide and phenothiazines are the commonest; among the others are cimetidine, haloperidol, methyldopa, pimozide and reserpine.
- Chronic renal failure and polycystic ovary syndrome are associated with mild elevations of prolactin.

Investigation

- *Slight to moderate elevation*—repeat the estimation, and if it is still elevated, screen for gross abnormality by lateral skull X-ray. If this shows enlargement of the pituitary fossa or erosion of the clinoid processes proceed to CT scan to detect a macroadenoma.
- *Marked elevation*—repeat the test but arrange X-ray and CT scan for as soon as possible. The patient who has headaches or a visual field defect requires urgent investigation.
- MRI scanning offers better resolution of small microadenomas but this is of little additional practical value (see below).
- An abnormal pituitary fossa may not be caused by a pituitary tumour but can be due to the *empty sella syndrome*. In this there is a congenital incompleteness of roof of the fossa and the subarachnoid space extends into the fossa. It is a benign condition.

Treatment
- Microadenomas tend to grow slowly if at all. In up to 30% of patients spontaneous regression of microadenomas will occur.
- The treatment of choice is a dopamine agonist (e.g. bromocriptine, or cabergoline). This will suppress prolactin secretion (aim at levels of 200–300 mU/L), correct oestrogen deficiency, permit ovulation and reduce the size of most prolactinomas.
- Surgery and radiotherapy are usually reserved for patients with very large tumours with extrasellar manifestations (e.g. pressure on the optic chiasma).

If pregnancy ensues check visual field perimetry every 2 months and prescribe a dopamine agonist and seek specialist help if there is evidence of tumour re-growth.

Weight loss-associated amenorrhoea
- A loss of more than 10 kg is frequently associated with amenorrhoea. It usually occurs in young women (frequently teenagers); they become obsessed with their body image and starve themselves. Anorexia nervosa is a misnomer because there is no loss of appetite.
- Oestrogen levels can be profoundly suppressed. If a progestogen challenge test (see below) is negative, there is a significant risk of osteoporosis, and hormone replacement therapy should be given.
- Hypothalamo-pituitary-ovarian function is usually restored when the lost weight is regained but occasionally may take many months for normal cyclical activity to return and for amenorrhoea to resolve.
- Ovulation induction is not indicated unless the patient wishes to become pregnant.

Kallman's syndrome
- A rare cause of hypogonadotrophic hypogonadism in which anosmia is associated with primary amenorrhoea. The underlying cause is an absence of LHRH.
- Treatment with ethinyl oestradiol will induce normal secondary sexual development but the initial dosage should be low (<5 µg daily) to prevent premature epiphyseal fusion of long bones and arrest of breast development.
- Pulsatile LHRH therapy is a specific and reliable treatment for later ovulation induction.

'Post-pill amenorrhoea'
- The oestrogen/progestogen contraceptive pill does not predispose to amenorrhoea once pill-taking ceases.
- An assumption that amenorrhoea is merely an after-effect of pill-taking means that hyperprolactinaemia will be missed in one

case from five and premature ovarian failure in one case from ten.

- Once other underlying causes are excluded this type of amenorrhoea responds well to ovulation induction with clomiphene if pregnancy is desired.

BASIC INVESTIGATION OF AMENORRHOEA

- Check serum prolactin level and thyroid function.
- If a chromosomal anomaly is likely on clinical grounds (e.g. short stature), check the karyotype.
- Carry out a progestogen challenge test (e.g. medroxyprogesterone acetate 5 mg daily for 5 days) to check endogenous oestrogen levels. The occurrence of withdrawal bleeding shows that the endometrium is reactive and the outflow tract patent.
- If the prolactin level is normal, and there is no galactorrhoea, further investigation for a pituitary tumour is unnecessary. Galactorrhoea requires evaluation of the pituitary regardless of prolactin levels or menstrual pattern.
- If the prolactin level is significantly elevated a pituitary tumour must be excluded as described above.
- If bleeding does not follow a progestogen challenge, measure follicle stimulating hormone (FSH) and luteinising hormone (LH).
  —A low LH (<5 i.u./L) suggests hypogonadotrophic hypogonadism
  —A high FSH (>40 i.u./L) on successive readings indicates ovarian failure. If the woman is under 35 years of age check her karyotype. (The presence of a Y chromosome suggests that the risk of gonadal malignancy is high)
  —A low FSH and LH (<3 i.u./L) suggest constitutionally delayed puberty or hypothalamic amenorrhoea
  —A raised LH (>10 i.u./L) and normal FSH suggest polycystic ovary syndrome (see below).

OLIGOMENORRHOEA

Definition
The occurrence of menses on only five or fewer occasions per year.

Its causes are the same as those for secondary amenorrhoea, and if investigation is needed it should follow the same plan.

POLYCYSTIC OVARY SYNDROME (PCOS)

Definition
The association of hyperandrogenism with chronic anovulation in women without specific underlying diseases of the adrenal or pituitary glands.

There is evidence of an autosomal dominant mode of inheritance. The male phenotype may be premature balding.

Prevalence: PCOS is present in:
• 30–40% of women with amenorrhoea
• 75–90% of women with oligomenorrhoea
• >70% of women with anovulatory infertility.

Polycystic ovaries have also been found in:
• 20% of asymptomatic women (although the incidence of irregular menses and slight hirsutism was greater in this group— see Further Reading)
• up to 90% of hirsute women with regular menses.

Clinical features (roughly in order of frequency)
—Subfertility	—Acne/male pattern alopecia
—Hirsutism	—Family history of maturity onset
—Oligomenorrhoea	diabetes
—Obesity	—Recurrent miscarriage.
—Dysfunctional uterine bleeding	

• The menstrual disturbance often begins at the menarche, which may be delayed.
• The presence of pigmented velvety patches in the skin flexures and on the neck (*acanthosis nigricans*) in women with PCOS is associated with insulin resistance.

Diagnosis and differential diagnosis
• The diagnosis is usually based on a combination of clinical, ultrasonographic and biochemical criteria.
• High-resolution transvaginal ultrasound will show the morphological feature of polycystic ovaries (multiple peripheral follicles <8 mm diameter and prominent echo-dense stroma) in up to 80% of anovulatory women.
• If a woman has oligomenorrhoea, PCOS is likely in the presence of hirsutism, polycystic ovaries on ultrasound and excess circulating androgens.
• The differential diagnosis includes hyperprolactinaemia, acromegaly, congenital adrenal hyperplasia or androgen-secreting tumours of the ovary.

ENDOCRINE ABNORMALITIES
• Mean serum LH levels are usually increased, though normal concentrations do not exclude PCOS as LH release is pulsatile; FSH levels are normal.
• Serum concentrations of testosterone and androstenedione are raised in over 90% of cases.
• Serum concentrations of oestradiol (total and free) are within normal limits in early and mid-follicular phases. However the

pattern of secretion is abnormal with no pre-ovulatory or midluteal increase. These effects may be compounded in obese women due to peripheral conversion of androgens by adipose tissue.

METABOLIC ABNORMALITIES

Women with PCOS have a greater frequency and degree of hyperinsulinaemia and insulin resistance.

Pathogenesis

One suggested mechanism by which PCOS develops or continues is as follows.

- Insulin resistance may be the primary defect inherited or acquired due to insulin receptor antibodies. A small proportion may be due to primary abnormalities of adrenal androgen production (e.g. 21-hydroxylase deficiency).
- The resulting hyperinsulinaemia leads to amplification of the stromatrophic effect of LH on the ovary, a small effect at the pituitary level increasing the production of LH, and a direct hepatic action which reduces sex hormone-binding globulin (SHBG) production.
- The enhanced LH activity leads to an imbalance in ovarian steroidogenesis, with increased production of androgen (predominantly androstenedione and testosterone) by theca cells.
- Conversion of androgen to oestrogen within the follicle by granulosa cells is greatly reduced because of a *relative* deficiency of FSH, and the excess enters the circulation.
- Aromatisation of the androgen surplus occurs peripherally in adipose tissue independently of FSH. This leads to a relatively constant oestrogen production with a larger than usual proportion of oestrone.
- Acyclic formation of oestrogen, particularly when unopposed by progesterone, results in abnormal feedback on the pituitary. FSH is suppressed and LH secretion promoted.
- The altered gonadotrophin profile distorts ovarian steroidogenesis further by accentuating theca cell hyperfunction and suppressing granulosa cell aromatase activity.
- The extent to which hirsutism occurs depends on the intracellular conversion of androgens to the active dihydrotestosterone by 5α-reductase.
- Oligomenorrhoea may occur, but otherwise the unopposed action of oestrogen leads to dysfunctional bleeding.

Management of anovulation

- If the woman is obese, loss of weight may be all that is necessary.

- Cycle control can be achieved by a low-dose combined oral contraceptive pill if she does not wish to conceive.
- Ovulation can usually be induced with clomiphene but 20–25% of women do not respond. A 'low dose' schedule of gonadotrophins may be successful in these women (see p. 210).
- Treatment with HMG or pulsatile LHRH have been disappointing, but HMG following pituitary suppression with an LHRH analogue may be more successful.
- Low-dose FSH given subcutaneously by infusion pump may allow follicular maturation and, therefore, ovulation.
- Laparoscopic ovarian diathermy or laser 'drilling' should be reserved for cases which have not responded to drug treatment or in which the size of the ovaries is causing symptoms (see p. 210).
- Dysfunctional bleeding will usually respond to the combined oestrogen-progestogen pill or a progestogen only. This treatment will also reduce the increased risk of endometrial carcinoma occurring in these women due to prolonged unopposed oestrogen action.

Management of hyperandrogenism
See under 'Hirsutism' below.

Management of metabolic disorders
- Because of the increased risk of type II diabetes and cardiovascular disease:
  —carry out a glucose tolerance test, lipid profile in obese young women with PCOS
  —encourage weight reduction
  —also commence surveillance of blood pressure.
- These should be considered even in non-obese women with PCOS although there is, as yet, no evidence of benefit.

HIRSUTISM

Definition
Excessive and inappropriate growth of facial and body hair, usually with a male pattern of distribution.

The most important causes are:
- endocrine—PCOS; adrenal hyperplasia/Cushing's syndrome; hypothyroidism; acromegaly
- androgen-secreting tumours of adrenal or ovary
- drugs—e.g. androgens, anabolic steroids, danazol, diazoxide, phenytoin
- idiopathic.

Investigations aim to differentiate among the above potential causes.

TREATMENT
- Sympathetic handling and reassurance are necessary at all times
- Treat specific underlying conditions
- *Cosmetic treatment*: may be sufficient if hirsutism is moderate or localised
- *Antiandrogens*:
  —a combination of ethinyl oestradiol 35 µg with cyproterone acetate (CPA) 2 mg ('Dianette') is effective. It also provides contraception
  —potency is increased by adding CPA 25–50 mg/day for the first 10 days of each packet
  —improvement in hirsutes is slow, with maximal effect around 18 months. Treatment should be continued for at least 6 months
  —liver dysfunction is a rare but serious complication
  —spironolactone (with a low-dose oral contraceptive pill) is a less effective alternative used in the USA where CPA is not generally available.
- *Glucocorticoids*: dexamethasone (also combined with an oral contraceptive pill) can be used for women with excess adrenal androgens.

EXCESSIVE MENSTRUAL LOSS

- Normal menstruation is defined as that occurring every 21–35 days, lasting 2–7 days and resulting in the loss of between 35 and 40 ml of blood.
- Excessive loss can be due to menses which are too long, too frequent, too heavy, and/or too irregular.
- 'Menorrhagia' is defined as 'excessive' (80 ml or more) regular menstrual loss.
- Objective measurement of loss is not routinely practicable.

CAUSES

Physiological
Menorrhagia is a subjective complaint which might not be confirmed if blood loss were to be measured in all cases. About 30% of women describe their menstrual loss as heavy. In a study measuring menstrual loss, 25% of women with loss <60 ml considered that they had heavy menses; 40% of women with loss >80 ml considered that they had normal menses.

Dysfunctional uterine bleeding (DUB—60% of cases)
- This is defined as *excessive menstrual loss not due to organic disease*.
- DUB can occur during *anovulatory cycles* in which a prolonged cycle usually ends in heavy, persistent vaginal bleeding.

—Anovulation is commonest at the extremes of menstrual life
—The older women who develop it are often obese (see below) and it is commoner when carbohydrate intolerance (e.g. maturity onset diabetes) is present
—It can occur as part of the polycystic ovary syndrome
—It may be associated with other endocrine disorders, e.g. hypothyroidism, adrenal hyperplasia, acromegaly.
- The proliferative effects of oestrogen are unopposed by progesterone.
    —The hyperplastic endometrium is shed when the ovarian follicle begins to degenerate or the endometrium outgrows its blood supply
    —In its most severe form there is *cystic glandular hyperplasia* of the endometrium and the clinical result is known as *metropathia haemorrhagica*.
- DUB occurring during *ovulatory cycles* is related to local disorders of prostaglandins and their receptors in the endometrium.
- Characteristically heavy regular menses occur in a 35- to 45-year-old woman, often accompanied by lower abdominal discomfort, dysmenorrhoea and dyspareunia. The uterus is slightly enlarged and can be markedly tender to palpation.
- The endometrium is normal.

Other gynaecological causes (35% of cases)
- *Endometriosis*—see page 197
- *Chronic pelvic inflammatory disease*—see page 230
- *Uterine tumours*, e.g. submucous leiomyomas (see p. 277); carcinoma of the endometrium (see p. 280) may develop in cases of pre-existing endometrial hyperplasia
- *Ovarian theca cell and granulosa cell tumours* often produce oestrogen (see p. 288) and cause menorrhagia
- *Intrauterine devices* (IUDs). The menstrual loss doubles in up to 50% of IUD users.

Endocrine and haematological causes (<5% of cases)
- Thyroid disorders
- von Willebrand's disease and idiopathic thrombocytopenia (or rarely leukaemia) may present with menstrual disorders. Women on long-term anticoagulant therapy may have menorrhagia
- Post-sterilisation: there is no convincing evidence that menstrual loss increases after sterilisation
- Psychological factors can play an important part.

MANAGEMENT OF EXCESSIVE MENSTRUAL LOSS
INVESTIGATION
- A comprehensive history and examination is vital.

- A menstrual diary collected over several months can be helpful.
- Take blood for full blood count and film and check thyroid function and glucose tolerance as necessary.
- Endometrial sampling should be carried out in women of 40 years of age or over. It is rarely necessary (or useful) in younger women. If possible it should be carried out as an outpatient procedure. **Note**: it is a diagnostic procedure which is virtually never therapeutic in even the short term.

GENERAL MANAGEMENT

- Specific organic disorders must be treated appropriately.
- The obese woman must be strongly advised to lose weight.
- Reassurance should be offered about normal levels of blood loss.

Drug treatment

- *Anovulatory cycles* will usually respond to progestogen therapy from day 15 (or earlier) to day 25 of the cycle. Young women can be given the combined oestrogen/progestogen pill.
- *Dysfunctional bleeding associated with ovulatory cycles* is much more difficult to manage in the long term:
  —the evidence suggests that antifibrinolytic therapy using tranexamic acid taken during menstruation is the most effective drug treatment. No increased risk of thromboembolism has been observed
  —*prostaglandin synthetase inhibitors* (e.g. mefenamic and flufenamic acids or naproxen sodium) are also effective
  —it is suggested that either of the above types of drug be considered as first line treatment
  —initial results using the *progestogen-releasing intrauterine device* are encouraging
  —*Progestogen* therapy is ineffective and has side-effects (e.g. nausea, breast tenderness, water retention)
  —*Ethamsylate* can reduce loss by reducing capillary fragility and inhibiting PG synthesis
  —*Danazol* reduces loss but has many androgenic and other unwanted side-effects.

Surgical treatment

It is important for the operator to have the appropriate training, skills and supervision.

- *Hysterectomy* is the most common surgical remedy:
  —about 80% are performed abdominally although the proportion carried out vaginally is increasing
  —laparascopically-assisted hysterectomy may be appropriate for some women but this needs to be evaluated further (see p. 299)
  —although there is no evidence of a need to remove healthy ovaries as a matter of routine (in women who are not at high

risk of ovarian cancer—see p. 291), oophorectomy (often bilateral) is carried out in up to 50% of abdominal hysterectomies
—the rate of post-operative infection can be significantly reduced by antibiotic prophylaxis.

- *Endometrial ablation* by Nd-YAG laser or resection under hysteroscopic control should be considered. The short-term advantages are not necessarily sustained in the long term. Table 16.1 compares them with hysterectomy (see 'Effective Health Care' in Further Reading).

Table 16.1 Endometrial ablation/resection: compared with hysterectomy

Outcome measure	Hysterectomy	Endometrial ablation/resection
Post-operative complications	Up to 45% for abdo.hyst— e.g. pain, haemorrhage wound infection, UTI (less for vag.hyst?): mortality 0.4–2/1000	<15%—uterine perforation, fluid overload, haemorrhage, UTI; mortality— anecdotal reports only
Effectiveness	100% have amenorrhoea	Amenorrhoea in 15–25%; light loss in further 60–75%
Return to normal activities (weeks)	from 4 to 12 weeks	from 1 to 4 weeks
Re-operation rate	nil	about 15% and 25% at 1 and 2 years respectively
'Satisfaction'	better in the medium to long term	no significant difference after 4 months
Comparative cost	higher initially	about 50% saving at 4 months but only 30% at 2 years

Endometrial hyperplasia

- If the glands and stroma increase together and there are no atypical cells the risk of developing malignancy is under 2%.
- If hysterectomy is not carried out initially such women should be kept under observation by annual outpatient endometrial sampling.
- If the hyperplasia is 'atypical' (with abnormal cells in irregular glands) the risk of endometrial adenocarcinoma is increased and hysterectomy is indicated (see p. 280).

DYSMENORRHOEA AND THE PREMENSTRUAL SYNDROME

PRIMARY DYSMENORRHOEA

Definition

Painful periods for which no organic or psychological cause can be found.

Features

- It usually occurs in teenage girls.
- The pain is colicky and usually begins shortly after or at the onset of menses.
- It tends to last for only 24–48 hours.
- There is often an exacerbating psychological element.
- There may be an increased production of prostaglandins. It occurs only in ovulatory cycles.

Management

- Exclude organic causes by history and examination.
- Suppression of ovulation using the combined oestrogen/progestogen pill may be helpful, or progestogens alone in the second half of the cycle.
- Symptomatic relief can often be obtained by prostaglandin synthetase inhibitors such as mefenamic and flufenamic acids or naproxen sodium.
- Procedures such as forced dilatation of the cervix or pre-sacral neurectomy are never indicated.

SECONDARY DYSMENORRHOEA

Definition

Painful periods for which an organic or psychosexual cause can be demonstrated.

Features

- It usually commences in adult life.
- It begins several days before the menses and gradually increases in severity as menses approach.
- The commonest associations are with pelvic inflammatory disease, endometriosis, fibroids or psychosexual problems.

Management

Laparoscopy can be helpful in ascertaining the cause, which can then be treated.

PREMENSTRUAL SYNDROME

A symptom complex of unknown aetiology occurring in the week before menstruation.

Features
- Most frequent around the age of 35 years.
- Tension, irritability and depression can be marked. 'Fluid retention' causes a bloated feeling in the abdomen, breast tenderness and swollen clumsy fingers.
- There is an increased susceptibility to accidents, criminal acts and suicide among women during the premenstrual phase.

Management
- Treatment is empirical because the cause is unknown. Placebo response is high.
- Sympathetic handling and understanding are of paramount importance.
- There have been few properly controlled trials of any of the many proposed remedies. Among them are the following:
    —*pyridoxine* (vitamin B$_6$) may provide some relief but this has not been clearly demonstrated in good trials
    —*evening primrose oil* contains prostaglandin precursors and may be of benefit
    —the *combined oral contraceptive pill* may help some women, though this has yet to be tested properly
    —trials of *progestogen* therapy (e.g. didrogesterone or progesterone) from mid-cycle have not shown clear benefit
    —empirical use of *diuretics* is not justified. They can be of benefit in some women who have oedema or measured weight increase (not merely bloating)
    —*luteinising hormone releasing hormones (LHRH) agonists plus oestrogen* may be useful for short-term treatment of severe cases.
- Hysterectomy and bilateral salpingo-oophorectomy may be necessary for a small group of women who are particularly severely affected.

ENDOMETRIOSIS

Definition
- The presence of endometrial tissue in sites other than the uterine cavity.
- In internal endometriosis (adenomyosis) the ectopic endometrium is confined to the myometrium.
- External endometriosis, with deposits occurring in a variety of ectopic sites, is more common but is seldom found together with adenomyosis. This argues for different aetiological factors.

EXTERNAL ENDOMETRIOSIS

Features
- The more 'endometriosis' is recognised the less well we seem to understand it!

—It is found in over 20% of asymptomatic women undergoing
   sterilisation (in whom it may be a normal physiological variant)
   —Clinically it presents most commonly in nulliparous women or
   those of low parity at between 30 and 45 years of age.
- The 'characteristic' symptoms are:
   —heavy, often irregular menses
   —secondary dysmenorrhoea (25–30%)
   —dyspareunia (30–40%)
   —pelvic pain between menses (40–60%)
   —subfertility—found in 15–60% of women undergoing
   diagnostic laparoscopy.
- There may also be symptoms relating to organs contiguous with
   the uterus.
- However, the frequency and severity of symptoms presumed to
   be caused by endometriosis do not correlate well with the extent
   or site of lesions: many women are asymptomatic.
- The American Fertility Society revised classification of
   endometriosis is as follows:

Table 16.2   The American Fertility Society revised classification of endometriosis

ENDOMETRIOSIS		*<1 cm*	*1–3 cm*	*>3 cm*
Peritoneum:	superifical	1	2	4
	deep	2	4	6
Ovary: R	superficial	1	2	4
	deep	4	16	20
Ovary: L	superficial	1	2	4
	deep	4	16	20

POSTERIOR	Partial	Complete
CUL-DE-SAC OBLITERATION	4	40

ADHESIONS		*<1/3 enclosure*	*1/3–2/3 enclosure*	*>2/3 enclosure*
Ovary: R	filmy	1	2	4
	dense	4	8	16
Ovary: L	filmy	1	2	4
	dense	4	8	16
Tube: R	filmy	1	2	4
	dense	1*	8*	16
Tube: L	filmy	1	2	4
	dense	1*	8*	16

* If the fimbriated end of the fallopian tube is completely enclosed, change the point
assignment to 16.

Stage I	Minimal	Score 1–5
Stage II	Mild	Score 6–15
Stage III	Moderate	Score 16–40
Stage IV	Severe	Score >40

Pathogenesis
There are several theories for the development of external endometriosis:
- *metaplasia*—both epithelial and stromal cells of the endometrium have a common precursor in the coelomic epithelium and adjacent mesenchyme. This could account for all abdominal and pelvic endometriosis, and the rare cases in the rectovaginal septum, umbilicus and canal of Nuck
- *retrograde menstruation* and implantation of viable cells on, for example, the ovaries and peritoneum of the pouch of Douglas
- *mechanical transplantation* into scars at the time of surgery, e.g. hysterectomy or hysterotomy. It very rarely follows caesarean section
- *venous or lymphatic 'metastasis'*. This (or metaplasia) could account for the rare pulmonary endometriosis.

It seems probable that not all cases arise in the same way.

Pathology
- The appearances of endometriosis may develop gradually from non-pigmented, 'atypical' lesions to the typical black 'powder-burn' lesions. The former may also be more active 'biochemically'.
- The ectopic endometrium menstruates, causing severe irritation, a sterile inflammatory reaction, and dense adhesions.
- The commonest sites in order of frequency are:
  —both ovaries (55%) which may show merely surface deposits or contain 'chocolate' cysts (containing old menstrual blood) of various sizes. These may arise by invagination of surface deposits or metaplasia of follicular or luteal cells
  —the posterior leaf of the broad ligament (35%)
  —the pouch of Douglas (35%) and uterosacral ligaments (30%).
- The rectum, urinary tract or lungs may occasionally be involved.
- Fertility can be compromised by tubal and ovarian damage and pelvic adhesions. High concentrations of prostaglandins and macrophages in the peritoneal fluid of affected women may also affect fertility. However, the association between mild endometriosis and subfertility is not fully explained.

Diagnosis
- It is often suspected after a careful history is taken.
- The presence of tender nodules on the uterosacral ligaments is also suggestive.
- Careful and thorough laparoscopy is essential for proper diagnosis, but the significance of the occasional tiny deposits on e.g. the ovaries or pouch of Douglas is disputed.
- For histological diagnosis both glandular and stromal tissue must be present.

Medical treatment
- The object is to suppress endogenous cyclical changes in oestrogen and progesterone to prevent menses.
- This can be achieved using:
  —continuous therapy with progestogen or the oral contraceptive pill for 6–9 months
  —danazol or gestrinone for 4–6 months—these have androgenic side-effects and must be discontinued if signs of virilisation develop
  —gonadotrophin-releasing hormone (GnRH) agonist—for no more than 6 months due to bone loss during therapy. This is reversible once treatment is ended.

Surgical treatment
- *Conservative surgery* by laparoscopy or laparotomy: small deposits can be diathermied, excised or vaporised using a CO_2 laser. Large chocolate cysts require excision.
- *'Radical' surgery* is reserved for women with severe symptoms which have failed to respond to lesser remedies or when continuing fertility is not an issue.
  —The preferred operation is hysterectomy and bilateral salpingo-oophorectomy with excision of as many other endometriotic lesions as possible.
  —Prior treatment with danazol or GnRH agonists may be worthwhile in severe cases.

ADENOMYOSIS

Islets of endometrial tissue, glands and stroma are found deep in the uterine wall, which responds by hyperplasia of muscle and fibrous tissue.

Features
- It tends to occur in older, multiparous women, in contrast to external endometriosis.
- The clinical presentation is:
  —increasingly severe menorrhagia
  —secondary dysmenorrhoea
  —gradually enlarging tender uterus.
- Symptomatically it is difficult to differentiate from uterine fibroids or dysfunctional bleeding.
- The uterus may be diffusely thickened or there may be localised swellings closely resembling leiomyomas.
- Adenomyosis is virtually impossible to diagnose definitely other than by histology after hysterectomy.

Treatment
Hysterectomy with conservation of ovaries (unless there are other indications for their removal).

STROMAL ENDOMETRIOSIS

- This rare condition acts more like a neoplasm than do other forms of endometriosis.
- Histologically, solid masses of cells resembling endometrial stroma are found in the endometrial wall, but other features of neoplasm are uncommon (e.g. mitoses are few and pleomorphism slight). It may be a form of a low-grade sarcoma.

Features
- The peak incidence is between the ages of 35 and 50 years.
- The condition does not regress on removal of the ovaries.
- Metastases do occur, but rarely.
- Clinically it may present with menorrhagia or postmenopausal bleeding and pelvic pain.
- It is usually diagnosed only after hysterectomy. The prognosis is usually good.

FURTHER READING

Brosens I (ed) 1993 Endometriosis. Clinical Obstetrics and Gynaecology 7:673–868

Eden J A 1991 Hirsutism. In: Studd J (ed) Progress in Obstetrics and Gynaecology 9:319–334. Churchill Livingstone, Edinburgh

Effective Health Care 1995 The Management of Menorrhagia. University of Leeds, Leeds

Fox R 1994 Polycystic ovarian disease and insulin resistance: pathophysiology and wider health issues. In: Studd J (ed) Progress in Obstetrics and Gynaecology 11: 341–351. Churchill Livingstone, Edinburgh

Franks S 1995 Polycystic ovary syndrome. New England Journal of Medicine 333:853–861

Rock J A 1995 Endometriosis: critical developments in understanding and management. International Journal of Gynecology & Obstetrics 50 (Suppl. 1):1–42

Shaw R W 1991 Treatment of endometriosis. In: Studd J (ed) Progress in Obstetrics and Gynaecology 9:273. Churchill Livingstone, Edinburgh

Wardle P G, Hull M G 1993 Is endometriosis a disease? Clinical Obstetrics and Gynaecology 7:673–685

17. Fertility and subfertility

FERTILITY IN THE FEMALE

THE HYPOTHALAMUS

Controls anterior pituitary function by substances secreted by cells within it and transported to the pituitary via the portal circulation.

- A single decapeptide neurotransmitter controls FSH- and LH-gonadotrophin-releasing hormone (GnRH). Its half-life is only a few minutes, and a continuous but pulsatile release occurs. Release is controlled by:
  —a long feedback loop due to circulating target gland hormones
  —a short feedback loop due to the effect of gonadotrophins on the hypothalamus
  —an ultrashort feedback by which it inhibits its own synthesis
  —a series of neurotransmitters such as serotonin, melatonin, noradrenaline and dopamine (see below).
- The hypothalamus exerts a tonic negative control on prolactin through the major *prolactin inhibitory factor*, dopamine.

THE PITUITARY GLAND

The pituitary is influenced by the hypothalamus via:
- Tonic and cyclic centres for the secretion of GnRH:
  —the tonic centre is situated in the medial basal hypothalamus
  —it is responsible for basal levels of gonadotrophin
  —oestradiol has a negative feedback effect on it and it is also dopamine-dependent
  —the cyclic centre lies in the pre-optic area in the anterior part of the hypothalamus
  —it is responsive to positive feedback by oestradiol and produces the mid-cycle surge of gonadotrophins:
- The posterior pituitary pathway:
  —cells in the supraoptic and paraventricular nuclei secrete vasopressin, oxytocin and neurophysin
  —they are transported along the pituitary stalk to the posterior pituitary where they are stored in axonal terminals
  —they also pass into the cerebrospinal fluid (CSF) and then to the portal system of the anterior pituitary
  —oxytocin is involved in gonadotrophin secretion.

GONADOTROPHIN RELEASE

- There are two pools, one released immediately it is synthesised and the other held in reserve.
- The rate of storage exceeds release, which makes the mid-cycle surge possible. (This is also the time when sensitivity to GnRH is greatest.)
- Oestradiol inhibits immediate release and increases storage. The effect is overcome by the positive feedback action of oestradiol on the cyclic centre.
- Low levels of progesterone increase release and storage after oestrogen priming. High levels of progesterone increase GnRH pulse frequency.
- The release of LH is pulsatile, and of FSH non-pulsatile.

REGULATION OF THE MENSTRUAL CYCLE

Recruitment of follicles (days 2–6)
- Initiation of follicular growth is independent of gonadotrophin stimulation.
- Follicles grow during infancy, ovulation, periods of anovulation, pregnancy and the menopause until the numbers are exhausted. For the vast majority of follicles growth is limited and atresia inevitable.
- As FSH levels increase, a group of follicles begins to grow further but the mechanism by which these follicles are chosen is unknown.
- The period of initial growth ends as oestrogen levels rise 7–8 days before the pre-ovulatory LH surge.

Selection of follicles (days 7–10)
- FSH stimulates follicular growth but also facilitates steroidogenesis by increasing the activity or number of LH receptors.
- Changes in hormonal levels are regulated by feedback mechanisms:
    —oestradiol inhibits FSH (negative feedback)
    —low levels of oestradiol inhibit LH
    —high levels of oestradiol stimulate LH (positive feedback) and FSH.

Dominant follicle selection (days 10–14)
- Oestrogens rise slowly, then rapidly, to peak just before ovulation.
- FSH fails due to negative feedback.
- LH increases steadily to its mid-cycle surge.
- The follicle destined to ovulate protects itself by its own hormone production. Ovarian stromal cell production of androgens (androstenedione and testosterone) increases,

enhancing the atresia of non-ovulatory follicles and stimulating libido.

Ovulation
- The rapid rise in oestrogen triggers an LH and FSH surge.
- The LH surge triggers resumption of meiosis by the oocyte.
- Degeneration of the collagen in the follicular wall allows it to rupture.
- Expulsion of the oocyte is brought about by prostaglandins induced by LH, and hormones such as noradrenaline and relaxin.
- The LH surge also triggers breakdown of the basement membrane between the theca and granulosa cell layers of the follicle wall.
- The granulosa layer is invaded by new blood vessels, exposing the cells to cholesterol for the first time in the cycle. This allows them to synthesise and secrete progesterone.

Luteal phase
- Days 1–3 post ovulation: granulosa cells increase in size, accumulate lutein (a yellow pigment) and secrete progesterone (see above).
- Days 8–9 post ovulation: peak level of progesterone is reached. (A plasma level of progesterone over 30 nmol/L (10 ng/ml) is good presumptive evidence of ovulation.)
- Days 9–11 post ovulation: the corpus luteum begins to decline unless pregnancy supervenes. Regression may be due to a local luteolytic effect or to oestradiol production by the CL. In pregnancy it is maintained by hCG until 6–8 weeks' gestation.
- In the absence of pregnancy the time from the LH surge to the onset of menstrual flow is usually 14 days.

FERTILITY IN THE MALE

The testes have two functions: *steroidogenesis* by the interstitial cells of Leydig between the seminiferous tubules; and *spermatogenesis*, which begins in the germinal epithelium of the tubules.

The seminiferous tubules and interstitial cells are controlled by:
- GnRH and gonadotrophins
- positive and negative feedback signals. Testicular steroids (particularly oestrogen) inhibit GnRH. Androgens diminish the LH-releasing effect of GnRH without affecting FSH. Oestrogen potentiates FSH and LH secretion by GnRH. Seminiferous tubules secrete *inhibin*, a non-steroid substance, which specifically inhibits FSH release.

The effects of androgens are:
- spermatogenesis
- development of accessory glands

- development of secondary sex characteristics
- metabolic and psychic effects determining 'maleness'
- increasing libido
- feedback on the hypothalamus and pituitary (see above).

ERECTION

Erection is due to tumescence of the penile cavernous bodies. It is mediated through the parasympathetic nervi erigentes (S2–4).

EJACULATION

Ejaculation is a reflex action involving a complex coordinated autonomic stimulation of the genital tract. It has two stages.
- Contractions of the epididymis, vas deferens and seminal vesicle pump sperm from the epididymis and seminal fluid from the prostate and seminal vesicles into the posterior urethra. As the seminal fluid arrives in the prostatic urethra contraction of the internal urethral sphincter closes the bladder neck (this prevents retrograde ejaculation). The second stage is triggered.
- The semen is expelled due to relaxation of the external sphincter and rhythmic contractions of ischiocavernous, bulbo-cavernous and perineal muscles.

TESTICULAR FUNCTION AND AGE

- Gonadal function in men is preserved well into old age and any decline is gradual.
- Although FSH and LH levels remain normal, testosterone levels tend to fall, suggesting decreased sensitivity to gonadotrophin.
- The so-called 'male climacteric' is more likely to be related to psychological, cardiovascular and neurological effects of ageing than to diminished production of androgens.

SUBFERTILITY

Definition
The involuntary failure to conceive within 12 months of commencing unprotected intercourse. Primary subfertility—no previous pregnancy; secondary subfertility—previous pregnancy (whatever the outcome).
- Incidence of primary subfertility alone is at least 12% of married couples.
- Causes (and approximate incidence):
  - —idiopathic   25%
  - —sperm defects or functional disorder   25%
  - —ovulation failure   20%
  - —tubal damage   15%
  - —endometriosis   5%

—coital failure	5%
—cervical mucus defect	3%
—azoospermia	2%

- Aims of investigation:
  —an explanation for the infertility
  —a prognosis
  —a basis for treatment.

Principles of management
- Deal with the infertile couple together.
- No one is 'at fault' or 'to blame'.
- Carry out investigations and treatments consistently in proper sequence.

INVESTIGATIONS

History
Check past medical, surgical and family histories.

Subfertility: investigations	
Both partners	Sexually transmitted disease
	Coital history
	Previous pregnancies
Female	Menstrual history
	Galactorrhoea
	Hirsutism
Male	Mumps orchitis
	Occupation—excess heat, radiation, toxic chemicals, sedentary job?

Examination
Female: look for signs of endocrine or other systemic diseases, hirsutism, tumours and genital abnormalities. Carry out general examination. Perform postcoital test (PCT) and cervical score (see below).

Male: look for signs of endocrine or other systemic diseases, lack of virilisation and genital abnormalities including testicular size, epididymal cysts and varicoceles.

ROUTINE INVESTIGATION IN THE FEMALE

General
Check for *Chlamydia* and rubella antibody levels. If the latter is negative, immunise and advise against pregnancy for 3 months.

Treat any possible chlamydial infection (see p. 230) especially *before* testing tubal patency.

Investigation of ovulation
- Basal body temperature recording (BBTR)
  —A temperature rise in mid-cycle sustained for about 14 days suggests that ovulation may have taken place, but it is not an accurate index of progesterone levels
  —The following features may suggest, but are not diagnostic of, abnormal ovulation patterns: monophasic (perhaps an inability to take temperature), slow rise in temperature, or short elevation of temperature.
- Serum progesterone—mid-luteal phase
- Endometrial biopsy if no hormone assays are available and to exclude tuberculosis where the disease is common
- Ovulation patterns vary between cycles and it may therefore be necessary to repeat tests on more than one occasion.

Postcoital test (see Tables 17.1, 17.2)
About 12 hours after intercourse, after 3–5 days' abstinence.

Normal (positive): more than 5 sperms with progressive motion per high-power field (HPF).

Inconclusive: 1–5 sperms with good motility.

Abnormal (negative): no sperm *or* all immobile/non-progressive *or* sperm agglutination.

For a valid inconclusive or abnormal result the cervical mucus must be pre-ovulatory—clear, copious (>0.3 ml), ductile (>10 cm) and pH >6.5.

Table 17.1 Evaluation of the cervical factor

PCT	Action
Normal	Cervix not implicated
No sperm	Sperm in vaginal pool?
	If no — psychosexual problem
	If yes — perform SIT/crossed penetration test
Sperm dead or clumped	Check for anti-sperm antibodies in wife
	Perform SIT/crossed penetration test
	Endocervical swabs for routine organisms and *Neisseria, Mycoplasma* or *Chlamydia*

SIT = sperm invasion test. .

Table 17.2

Causes of abnormal SIT	Treatment
Endocervicitis	Antibiotics Cryocautery to cervix
Failure of cervix to respond to endogenous oestrogen	Ethinyl oestradiol 50 µg daily for 10 days from start of cycle and repeat PCT. A positive result is an indication for gonadotrophin therapy. If negative, consider assisted conception (p. 214)
Anti-sperm antibodies in semen or mucus	Steroid therapy is of no proven benefit and may cause severe side-effects. Selected cases may benefit from IVF with specific sperm-preparation techniques to remove the antibodies.

Hysterosalpingography (HSG)

Indications
- History/examination suggest tubal damage, or if chlamydial antibody titres are elevated
- Other investigations abnormal or infertility persists despite treatment
- Previous surgery on uterus or tubes.

The woman must avoid pregnancy in HSG cycle. General anaesthetic is seldom necessary. Buscopan i.v. can be given to counteract tubal spasm.

ROUTINE INVESTIGATION IN THE MALE

Semenalysis
Test after 3 days' abstinence from intercourse. Three readings 1 month apart are necessary to confirm abnormality.
- Normal values:
  —volume 2–6 ml
  —density $20–250 \times 10^6$ ml
  —motility >50% with forward motion within 2 hours
  —morphology >50% normal sperm.
- Other features to be noted:
  —viscosity   —liquefaction
  —sperm clumping   —presence of inflammatory cells.
- Anti-sperm antibodies can be tested for, using the *mixed erythrocyte-spermatozoa antiglobulin reaction* (MAR test). Anti-Rh antibodies and semen are mixed with Rh-positive erythrocytes. If spermatozoa carry anti-sperm antibodies they are caught up in the agglutination reaction.

FURTHER MANAGEMENT IN THE FEMALE

Induction of ovulation

- Defective ovulation can be due to:
  —non-specific hypothalamo-pituitary dysfunction
  —hyperprolactinaemia
  —polycystic ovarian disease (see p. 188)
  —other endocrine disorders.
- The cumulative conception rate after 2 years is 95% for amenorrhoeic women and 80% for those with oligomenorrhoea (when these are the sole disorders).

Amenorrhoeic women

If the patient is amenorrhoeic with normal prolactin and gonadotrophin levels, carry out a progestogen challenge test.

- If no withdrawal bleeding follows Provera 5 mg daily for 5 days, gonadotrophin or pulsatile GnRH therapy is likely to be necessary.
- If withdrawal bleeding occurs, therapy with oral fertility agents is indicated (see below).

Women having menstrual cycles (however irregular)

- If mid-luteal progesterone levels are low, prescribe clomiphene or tamoxifen (see below).
- Check progesterone levels again in the second treatment cycle. If normal ovulation is still not occurring, the dose of clomiphene or tamoxifen can be increased.
- If there is still no ovulation, check plasma oestrogen levels and/or follicular growth using ultrasound in the follicular phase.
- A good rise in oestrogen or follicular growth without ovulation, or failure of any oestrogen response or follicular growth, suggests that gonadotrophin therapy is likely to be necessary.
- If pregnancy does not occur within six treatment cycles despite good ovulation, review other factors critically (but continue therapy).

Oral fertility agents

These compete with natural oestrogens by blocking receptors in target organs, including the pituitary, leading to increased FSH levels. Follicles develop and ovulation follows in 85% of well-oestrogenised women.

- *Clomiphene.* The dose is 50–150 mg daily from days 2 to 6 or days 5 to 9 of the cycle. Side-effects are few: visual disturbances may occur.
- *Tamoxifen.* The dose is 10–40 mg twice daily for 5 days as above. Side-effects are few.

The incidence of miscarriage and twins is slightly increased. Ovarian hyperstimulation is rare and usually resolves spontaneously.

Laparoscopic ovarian diathermy

The minimal access surgical equivalent of ovarian wedge resection. The mechanism of action is not well understood.

- This treatment is appropriate only for women with polycystic ovarian syndrome (see p. 188) *and* who are unresponsive to clomiphene, have early follicular phase serum LH levels >10 i.u./L *or* who recurrently respond excessively to gonadotrophin therapy.
- With laser, the multiple small subcapsular follicles are ruptured giving a 'pepperpot' appearance to the ovarian surface.
- With diathermy, the central stromal tissue of the ovary is partially destroyed by inserting the diathermy needle at several sites.
- LH levels fall after treatment and ovulation will occur spontaneously in about 75–80% of treated women for up to 9 months. This offers the chance of natural conception.
- The remaining 20–25% of women will either become responsive to clomiphene or have a more predictable response to gonadotrophins.
- About 15% of patients may develop peri-ovarian adhesions.

Gonadotrophin therapy

This is indicated in women with hypogonadotrophic hypogonadism who are resistant to oral agents or pulsatile GnRH.

- Occasional and casual use is dangerous because:
  —ovarian sensitivity varies between cycles and patients
  —the difference in dose between normal ovulation and hyperstimulation is small
  —the rate of multiple conceptions and miscarriage is high unless control is meticulous.
- Human menopausal gonadotrophin (HMG) or purified FSH is used to stimulate follicular development.
- Women who have hypothalamic or hypopituitary causes of ovulation failure (e.g. Kallman's syndrome) will require HMG for an adequate response because it contains both LH and FSH.
- After follicular development has been stimulated, human chorionic gonadotrophin (HCG) induces ovulation.
- Treatment should be monitored by serial serum oestradiol assays and ultrasound measurement of follicular growth (number and size).

Multiple pregnancy rate Between 12 and 45% depending on the degree of control. If good, 75% of the multiple pregnancies are twins. *Anything higher is a failure of treatment.*

Hyperstimulation Mild in 6% of cases—excess oestrogen output with ovarian enlargement; no cysts; some abdominal pain. No active treatment is needed. *Moderate*—detectable but not large ovarian cysts; abdominal pain, nausea, vomiting, diarrhoea and ascites. Admit for observation, rehydration and symptomatic treatment. Infusion of colloid (intravenous albumin) may be necessary. *Severe* (2% of cases)—large ovarian cysts, massive ascites (possibly with hydrothorax). Severe abdominal pain and distension. There is a risk of DIC and thromboembolism if the woman has an underlying thrombophilic tendency (see p. 303).

Management Correct fluid and electrolyte imbalance (avoid diuretics). Intravenous colloid should be used for infusion rather than crystalloid. Screen for early evidence of DIC. Laparotomy only if cysts have ruptured or are bleeding.

Gonadotrophin-releasing hormone (GnRH or LHRH)
- Pulsatile subcutaneous (or intravenous) infusion of GnRH by miniaturised automatic infusion systems is indicated mainly for ovulation induction in women with hypothalamic or hypopituitary causes of ovulation failure.
- It can also be successful in treatment-resistant hyperprolactinaemia and clomiphene-resistant anovulation.
- Endocrine events in the normal cycle are mimicked and the multiple pregnancy rate is low.
- Treatment is monitored using ultrasound measurement of follicular development.
- After ovulation the pulsatile infusion may be discontinued and luteal phase support may be given by a single injection of hCG.
- It is usually ineffective in women with polycystic ovary syndrome (PCOS—see p. 188).

TUBAL FACTORS
- HSG and laparoscopy (with or without hysteroscopy) are complementary investigations of tubal function.
- Ultrasound assessment of tubal patency is now possible but gives no information about damage to the endosalpinx. As this is an important predictor for success of tubal microsurgery, HSG is preferred.

Indications for laparoscopy
- Abnormal HSG.
- History or examination suggest need for direct investigation, e.g. endometriosis.
- All other investigations normal, or abnormal but corrected (in such cases unsuspected problems can be found in up to 30%).

Peritubal adhesions Avascular adhesions can be divided at laparoscopy or laparotomy (salpingolysis). Treatment of vascular adhesions gives poor results.

Tubal blockage Micro-surgery for mild/moderate damage, IVF if severe.

Salpingostomy Surgical opening of ostia. Conception rate no more than 20%.

Excision of block and re-anastomosis—conception rate 10–15%.

- The incidence of ectopic pregnancies is increased in treated cases.

FURTHER MANAGEMENT IN THE MALE

Erectile impotence
Among the causes are psychosexual problems, vascular disease (e.g. secondary to smoking) and hyperprolactinaemia.

Causes of azoospermia
Ejaculatory failure

- Exclude retrograde ejaculation by examining urine postcoitally (especially if ejaculate volume <2 ml).
- If psychogenic impotence is present, refer for psychosexual counselling.
- Consider neurological disorders (e.g. multiple sclerosis or diabetic neuropathy), urological factors and drug side-effects (e.g. antihypertensive therapy).

Failure of spermatogenesis

- Assess testicular size—this diagnosis is more likely if volume <15 ml by orchidometer
- Check FSH levels. Significant elevation is found in:
  —Klinefelter's syndrome (therefore check karyotype)
  —spermatogenic arrest
  —Sertoli cell only syndrome
  —testicular atrophy.
- In selected cases intracytoplasmic sperm injection (ICSI) may be possible; but there is no remedy in the majority of cases.

Obstruction

If testicular size and consistency and FSH are normal, consider congenital or acquired block of the vasa by semen biochemistry (see below) and/or vasography.

Hypogonadotrophism

- This is indicated by lack of virilisation, impotence and reduced testosterone level with normal or low FSH and LH levels.
- It is the only treatable cause of azoospermia using HMG. Because spermatogenesis takes over 70 days, treatment must be prolonged. Once spermatogenesis has been stimulated HCG alone will maintain sperm counts.

Oligospermia

- This is often accompanied by seminal plasma of high viscosity and/or low volume which fails to liquefy.

- Low sperm density and poor motility are frequently related.
- Seminal biochemistry (see Table 17.3) may indicate the source of the problem.

Table 17.3 Seminal biochemistry

Acid phosphatase, zinc	Fructose	Carnitine	Possible site of defect
Absent	Present	Present	Prostate
Present	Absent	Present	Seminal vesicles
Present	Present	Absent	Epididymis

- Elevated FSH levels (<8 i.u./L) suggest irreversible sterility. Low levels of testosterone and high LH levels are frequently secondary to severe testicular damage which is irreversible.
- Testicular biopsy is of little diagnostic value.
- *Cytogenetic studies.* Karyotype will reveal abnormalities in up to 6% of infertile males and 20% when azoospermia is present. No treatment is available apart from donor insemination (DI).
- *Therapy for oligospermia.* There is no proven effective drug treatment. All claims for success using clomiphene or mesterolone must be compared with the spontaneous pregnancy rate in oligospermic men. High ligation of a varicocele improves semenalysis in 60% of cases but is of no proven benefit for conception.

Artificial insemination
- Husband (AIH)—only when intercourse is impossible due to male impotence or anatomical defects but a normal ejaculate can be obtained
- Donor insemination (DI)—the greatest care must be taken to:
  —protect the identity of the donors
  —ascertain that both husband and wife are sure they wish this form of treatment. Inseminations are usually carried out twice in the peri-ovulatory phase. Prior investigation of female infertility is mandatory. Checking for stress-induced ovulatory dysfunction during the initial 2–3 treatment cycles is advisable.

Intracytoplasmic sperm injection (ICSI)
- Individually selected sperm are injected into oocytes by microscopic manipulation before in vitro fertilisation (IVF).
- It is appropriate for men with severe oligospermia or significant sperm dysfunction.
- In conjunction with surgical recovery of sperm from the epididymis or testis, it can also by-pass the problem for men with:
  —congenital absence of the vas (exclude an association with carriage of the cystic fibrosis gene)

—failed reversal of vasectomy

—failed surgery for bilateral obstruction of the vas deferens.

- Follicular stimulation and oocyte collection from the woman is as for standard IVF (see below). Only morphologically mature oocytes are suitable for micro-injection.
- Under an operating microscope, the cumulus cells are removed chemically from the oocyte which is then held gently by a micro-pipette.
- A fine micro-pipette is used to draw up a single motile sperm (tail first). This is then advanced through the zona pellucida and vitelline membrane.
- The sperm is deposited (head first) into the cytoplasm of the oocyte nucleus.
- About 10% of sperm will be damaged by the procedure but fertilisation rates of 60–75% are now being reported.
- Pregnancy rates of up to 35% per cycle can be achieved after transfer of up to three embryos.
- ICSI is likely to reduce the demand for DI, currently the only alternative for many couples suffering from severe male subfertility.

ASSISTED CONCEPTION

These procedures are carefully controlled in the UK by the statutory Human Fertilisation and Embryology Authority (HFEA).

In vitro fertilisation (IVF)

- It is now estimated that up to 35% of subfertile couples could benefit from IVF.
- It is most suitable for women with tubal blockage or damage, endometriosis, or those with unexplained subfertility.
- The advent of ICSI now makes IVF appropriate for treatment of male subfertility.
- IVF (or GIFT (gamete intrafallopian transfer)) may be used for egg donation and may optimise the chances of pregnancy for women over 35 years of age who have ovulatory disorders but have failed to conceive with gonadotrophin therapy.
- It is expensive and requires sophisticated laboratory facilities and highly skilled medical, nursing, scientific and technical personnel.

SUGGESTED GUIDELINES FOR PROCEEDING WITH ASSISTED CONCEPTION

- Clear positive recommendation from GP
- No more than one previous child
- A continuing stable heterosexual relationship of at least 2 years' duration

- Treatment is technically feasible with a good chance of success, e.g. not in women of 40 years or over?
- Couples in good health such that they can be reasonably expected to bring up the child together
- Appropriate domestic and social circumstances
- An understanding by all parties of the statutory responsibility to consider the welfare of any child born as a result of treatment.

(*These guidelines could, in fact, be applied to the whole problem of infertility.*)

OUTLINE PROTOCOL FOR IVF

- Multiple ovulation is induced with HMG or purified FSH after pituitary down-regulation with a GnRH analogue to inhibit any endogenous LH rise. Follicular maturation is monitored ultrasonically and by serum oestradiol levels.
- Mature oocytes are recovered just before ovulation (following an injection of hCG) by transvaginal aspiration of follicles under ultrasound guidance using i.v. sedation. Alternatively, laparoscopy may be used. The aim is to collect at least four eggs.
- Fertilisation of ovum by sperm occurs within 24 hours in a fluid culture medium at physiological temperature and atmospheric conditions. There is a 70% chance of each mature egg being fertilised.
- A legal maximum of three embryos are transferred to the uterus through the cervical canal after 2 to 3 days (i.e. around the eight-cell stage).

Gamete intra-fallopian transfer (GIFT)
- GIFT is suitable for all women who are candidates for IVF except those with blocked or damaged fallopian tubes, or when ICSI is used.
- Oocytes are collected as above, mixed with $2–5 \times 10^5$ sperm in buffered medium and transferred into the fimbrial end of the tube by laparoscopy.
- GIFT is theoretically superior to IVF because fertilisation occurs in the normal site and implantation at the normal time (5–6 days) after ovulation (cf. IVF at 2 days). This is reflected in the greater number of pregnancies and births with GIFT than in IVF (see below). It too is expensive, and the conditions for setting it up should be as for IVF.

Intrauterine insemination (IUI)
- IUI using partner's semen after superovulation of the woman can be useful in some cases.
- As with GIFT, it is only suitable for women with patent, healthy fallopian tubes.

- When used appropriately about 20% of the women will become pregnant and 15% will have a child.

Ovum donation followed by IVF
This can be used with the same considerations as for DI (p. 213) in women who:
- have had their ovaries removed
- have experienced premature menopause
- carry a serious genetic defect.

Appropriate hormonal support is required for the first two of these.

Results of IVF and GIFT
- Transfer of a single embryo results in a pregnancy in less than 10% of cases.
- It is therefore usual to transfer three embryos if possible. This gives a 25–30% chance of a single pregnancy, a 5% chance of twins, and a 1–2% chance of triplets.
- The overall efficiency of the method (the 'take-home baby rate') is between 15 and 20% for each cycle. This probably does not differ significantly from conception rates in normal couples.
- About 20% of women will have a child per cycle of IVF treatment compared with about 30% for GIFT.

FURTHER READING

Behrman S J, Patton G W, Holtz G (eds) 1994 Progress in infertility, 4th edn. Little, Brown, Boston
Fishel S (ed) 1994 Ballière's Clinical Obstetrics and Gynaecology 8: Micromanipulation techniques
Templeton A A, Drife J O (eds) 1992 Infertility. Springer Verlag, Berlin

18. Contraception and sterilisation

- Human fertility can be measured in several ways, e.g.:
  - *general fertility rate*—this is the number of births during a year per 1000 women of childbearing age
  - *age-specific fertility rate*—the number of births during a year per 1000 women of a specified 5-year age range
  - *total fertility rate*—the average size of a completed family.
- The '*Pearl index*' is a measure of contraceptive effectiveness using the numbers of pregnancies occurring per 100 woman-years (w.y.) of exposure.

STEROIDAL CONTRACEPTION

Steroidal contraception has, as its basis, synthetic oestrogens and progestogens. The effect of any one combined oral contraceptive (COC) will depend on the balance of the oestrogen and progestogen it contains.
- The oestrogen in most pills is now ethinyl oestradiol using the lowest possible effective dose.
- The 'traditional' progestogens have been ethynodiol, levonorgestrel and norethisterone.
- The newer progestogens desogestrel (DSG), gestodene (GSD) and norgestimate bind more specifically to progesterone receptors and have less effect on sex hormone-binding globulin (SHBG) and high-density lipoprotein (HDL). They are thus less anti-oestrogenic and may reduce the risk of arterial disease. There is, however, some evidence (see Further Reading) that the risk of venous thromboembolism with DSG and GSD is twice that using 'traditional' progestogens (information about norgestimate is insufficient). This is discussed further below.

Mode of action
- Inhibition of ovulation due to negative feedback on the hypothalamo-pituitary-ovarian axis
- Induction of changes in cervical mucus, endometrium, myometrium and fallopian tubes which makes them hostile to sperm and unfavourable for ovum transplant and implantation.

TYPES OF STEROIDAL CONTRACEPTIVES

- *Combined oral contraceptives (COC)* are the most widely used:
  —'monophasic' (fixed dose) pills. Oestrogen and progestogen
  are taken in constant doses for 21 days followed by an interval
  of 7 days
  —'biphasic' and 'triphasic' preparations containing phased doses
  of oestrogen and progestogen which make it possible to
  'titrate' the dose to the individual woman in order to find the
  lowest dose of both hormones that will provide good cycle
  control, and fewest side-effects.
- *Continuous low-dose oral progestogens (POP)* have a good
  contraceptive effect provided they are taken regularly 3–4 hours
  before expected intercourse.
  —Ovulation is only inhibited in 40% of women, and the anti-
  fertility effect on cervical mucus (which wears off after 16–20
  hours) is important
  —Irregular menstruation is frequent but improves as use
  continues. Some patients develop amenorrhoea
  —An association with ectopic pregnancies is still in dispute. The
  POP may produce a genuine increase because of its effect on
  the fallopian tube, or it may be less effective in preventing
  ectopic than intrauterine pregnancies. Where possible the
  COC or injectable progestogen (which inhibits ovulation)
  should be used in those with a past history of ectopic
  pregnancy
  —Lactation is not inhibited by POP and there does not appear to
  be an effect on blood pressure. They are particularly suitable
  for lactating women, diabetics, those with contraindications or
  intolerance to oestrogen, and possibly those with a past
  history of venous thrombosis.
- *Injectable progestogens* given as intramuscular injections, for
  instance of medroxyprogesterone acetate (Depo-Provera)
  150 mg every 3 months or norethisterone oenanthate 200 mg
  every 8 weeks.
  —They are highly effective
  —Menstruation tends to be irregular and may be prolonged:
  amenorrhoea will supervene in about one third of users within
  1 year
  —Effects on glucose tolerance and plasma lipids are markedly
  less than those caused by COC. Occasionally there is some
  weight gain
  —There appears to be no effect on blood pressure or blood
  coagulability
  —No increased risk of carcinoma of breast, endometrium or
  cervix has been noted
  —Menstrual cycles and fertility return to normal within 6 months
  of the last injection
  —If used during lactation the quality and quantity of milk are

improved. Only a tiny quantity of steroid is ingested by the infant and as yet no adverse effects have been noted
—Do not use in an already pregnant woman.
- *Implants* avoid the 'first-pass' effect of the oral route. 'Norplant' delivers levonorgestrel in six subdermal capsules.
    —If inserted within 24 hours of the start of menstruation, no additional contraception is required
    —The capsules should be removed before the end of 5 years. Training in insertion and removal is required.

(See below for progestogen-containing IUDs.)

- *Postcoital preparations* e.g. ethinyl oestradiol 100 µg and levonorgestrel 500 µg taken within 72 hours of unprotected intercourse and repeated 12 hours later.
    —Nausea and vomiting are common
    —It is not recommended as a routine method but is useful as an emergency method, including following rape.

Efficacy
- Failure can be due to the method or the patient
- With older 'medium-dose' COC the Pearl index was <1/100 w.y.
- With modern 'low-dose' COC the rate is about 3/100 w.y.
- The POP has a failure rate of 2–3/100 w.y. (in older women it can be as low as 0.9)
- Injectable progestogens have a Pearl index of 0–0.4/100 w.y.

Non-contraceptive benefits of COC
- Less dysmenorrhoea and menorrhagia (and therefore less anaemia)
- Reduced risk of carcinoma of endometrium and ovary (by at least 50%); pelvic inflammatory disease; and benign breast disease
- Possible protective effect against fibroids and rheumatoid arthritis.

Possible adverse effects of COC
The risk/benefit balance must be weighed for each woman, taking into account the presence of risk markers.

Metabolic changes
- *Weight gain*—associated with pills containing levonorgestrel but not desogestrel (DSG) or gestodene (GSD).
- *Carbohydrate metabolism*—modern low-oestrogen and progestogen preparations produce minor effects on insulin secretion and little or no change in glucose tolerance. Significant glucose intolerance occasionally occurs in susceptible individuals, and insulin-dependent diabetics may need to increase their dose.
- *Lipid metabolism*. The effect on the ratios of total and low density lipoprotein (LDL) cholesterol to high density lipoprotein

(HDL) cholesterol (important indicators of risk of cardiovascular disease) depends on the relative doses of oestrogen/progestogen and the type of progestogen. The aim of modern pills is to have a near-neutral effect.

Table 18.1   Thrombotic and cardiovascular risks

Condition	Relative risk	Associated risk markers
Venous thrombosis	<2 with low-dose COC containing levonorgestrel, norethisterone or ethynodiol Pills containing DSG and GSD may increase that risk further × 2	Close family history; marked obesity (BMI >30 kg/m^2); immobility (e.g. plaster cast or in a wheelchair); prominent varicose veins; presence of factor V Leiden mutation
Haemorrhagic stroke	1.5–2	Smoking; hypertension
Thrombotic stroke: non-fatal fatal	5 in 1/10 000 w.y. in 2–4/10 000 w.y.	Close family history; smoking; diabetes; marked obesity
Hypertension	Develops in about 5% of women within 5 years of commencing COC: *stop if BP rises to 160/95 mmHg or more*	Age, family or personal history of hypertension; obesity and previous hypertension in pregnancy are not associated risks
Myocardial infarction: fatal	3–5 in 1/10 000 w.y.	Smoking, age, hypertension, hyperlipidaemia

Effects on gastrointestinal tract
Reports of an increased incidence of *cholelithiasis* and *cholecystitis* were associated with higher doses of oestrogen. The risk is not significantly increased with low-dose COC. A slight increased risk of ulcerative colitis and Crohn's disease is associated with COC use and smoking.

Cancer and COC use
• *Breast cancer:* COC use reduces the risk of benign breast disease but the question of an increased risk of breast cancer remains unresolved. Further studies are necessary on women at increased genetic risk of breast cancer and who use COC.

Studies suggesting an increased risk among young women (particularly if used before a first pregnancy) were conflicting and confusing. *If such a risk exists in these women it can be minimised by using the lowest effective doses of oestrogen and progestogen.*

- *Cervical neoplasia*: an increased incidence of *cervical intraepithelial neoplasia* is likely to be due to greater sexual activity in women on COC.

  There may be some slight direct effect of COC on *carcinoma of the cervix*, but this has to be set against the strongly protective effect against carcinoma of endometrium and ovary.

- *Ovarian cancer*. There is a >50% reduction and this effect persists for many years after stopping COC.
- *Endometrial cancer*: similarly reduced by at least 50%.

Drug interactions
- *Enzyme-inducing drugs* may reduce the effect of oestrogens and progestogens. They include most anticonvulsants (not sodium valproate), rifampicin and griseofulvin.
- *Interference with gut flora* and the enterohepatic circulation of ethinyl oestradiol can be caused by broad spectrum antibiotics (also by a vegetarian diet). Progestogens are not affected in this way.
- Advice depends on the length of therapy:
  —*short-term*—use barrier method during and for 7 days after stopping drug
  —*long-term*—use monophasic 50 μg ethinyl oestradiol COC (can be taken as four packs without a break then a 'tablet-free' interval): contraceptive efficacy can be judged by the occurrence of irregular bleeding.

CONTRAINDICATIONS TO COMBINED ORAL CONTRACEPTIVES

Absolute and relative contraindications are listed in the information boxes.

COC: absolute contraindications

Cardiovascular
- Previous arterial or venous thrombosis
- Ischaemic or other severe heart disease; pulmonary hypertension
- Coagulation tendency (e.g. activated protein C resistance due to factor V Leiden mutation) or blood dyscrasias
- Previous cerebral haemorrhage
- Severe hypertension
- Focal migraine; transient ischaemic attacks
- Hyperlipidaemia
- Combination of risk markers (see above)

Hepatic
- Chronic liver disease, and following acute disease until liver function tests have been normal for 3 months
- Cholestatic jaundice of pregnancy
- Chronic idiopathic jaundice (e.g. due to Dubin–Johnson or Rotor syndromes)
- Liver adenoma; porphyrias

Other
- Oestrogen-dependent neoplasms (particularly breast cancer)
- History of serious condition affected by sex steroids, e.g. pemphigoid gestationis; haemolytic uraemic syndrome
- Undiagnosed abnormal genital tract bleeding
- Pregnancy

COC: relative contraindications

- Oligomenorrhoea (investigate first and may then be prescribed if no other contraindication)
- Women over 35 years of age who smoke
- Latent or established diabetes
- Cholelithiasis (but can be used after cholecystectomy)
- First-degree relative with breast cancer
- Obesity, if associated with other risk factors
- Non-focal migraine when ergotamine is not required for treatment
- Sickle cell disease (injectable progestogen better). Sickle cell trait is not a contraindication
- Crohn's disease

Prescribing COC

The following guidelines have recently been suggested by the Margaret Pyke Centre (see also Further Reading).

- *Which oestrogen*? Use the lowest acceptable dose.
- *Which progestogen*? Because of a supposed increased risk of *venous* thromboembolism (TE), in October 1995 the Committee on Safety of Medicines (CSM) in the UK advised that:
  —COC containing DSG or GSD should not be used in women with risk markers for TE including obesity, varicose veins. (A previous history of TE is an absolute contraindication to COC use.)
  —COC containing DSG or GSD should only be used by women who are 'intolerant of other COCs' *and* who are prepared to accept the supposed increased risk of TE.

  Note: this was despite a possible lesser risk of arterial disease (heart attack or stroke—see above).

- 'Intolerance of other COCs' includes irregular bleeding, weight gain, acne or headaches.
- Among the other women for whom a DSG/GSD pill might be more suitable are:
  —those with a single risk marker for *arterial* disease (see above)
  —those aged 35 up to the menopause in the absence of all risk markers for venous or arterial disease.
- If a DSG/GSD pill is to be used:
  —it must be the patient's informed choice
  —all counselling and discussion must be clearly recorded in the casenotes.

Surgery and the COC pill

- Whether or not to stop the pill before major surgery is controversial (see Further Reading)
- With low-dose oestrogen pills the risk of postoperative TE is about 1% for pill users and 0.5% for non-pill users.
- This must be balanced against the risks of stopping the pill 4–6 weeks before surgery, the most important of which is unwanted pregnancy.
- The woman must be made aware of the above and, if the COC is stopped, adequate alternative contraception must be provided.
- THRIFT (see Further Reading) suggest that *without other risk markers* there is insufficient evidence either to routinely stop the pill before elective major surgery or use specific prophylaxis.
- Prophylaxis is advised for emergency surgery.

INTRAUTERINE DEVICES (IUDs)

- Now the second most common reliable and reversible method of preventing pregnancy

- The ideal IUD must be effective; easy to fit (with minimal discomfort); and should remain in the uterine cavity until the woman wishes it removed.

Types of IUD in common use
- Copper (Cu)-containing with surface areas of 200–375 mm^2
- Progestogen-releasing.

Mode of action
- 'Foreign body' reaction
- Copper ions affect tubal fluid, sperm transport and oocytes
- Progestogens make cervical mucus 'hostile' and thin the endometrium.

Efficacy
- The Pearl index of the 200 mm^2 Cu devices is 2–4/100 w.y.
- For the newest devices with 375 mm^2 of copper- or progestogen-releasing, this falls to <1/100 w.y.

Timing of insertion
- The best time is towards the end of menstruation but, if necessary, fitting can take place at any point in the cycle.
- Post-pregnancy side-effects, expulsion or perforation rates are no higher if inserted at 3–4 weeks than at 6 weeks.
- An IUD can be fitted at the time of suction termination of pregnancy but the optimum time may be 1–2 weeks later because the risk of perforation is less.
- Insertion of an IUD within 5 days of unprotected intercourse will act as a post-coital contraceptive.

POSSIBLE COMPLICATIONS AND SIDE-EFFECTS OF IUDs

- *Vaginal bleeding*—this is the commonest reason for removal.
  —With Cu-releasing devices menstrual loss may increase by 40–50%
  —With progestogen-releasing devices loss is reduced by 40–50% but intermenstrual spotting/bleeding occurs in up to 80% of women.
- *Pain*—some low abdominal pain or backache may follow insertion.
  —Rarely it is severe and the device may need to be removed
  —Dysmenorrhoea can be increased particularly if the woman is nulliparous.
- *Vaginal discharge*—may be temporary or persistent.
  —It arises from the endometrium as it reacts to the presence of a foreign body but symptomatic discharges must be investigated.
- *Ectopic pregnancy*—the rate for modern IUDs is <1.5/1000 w.y.
  —Cu-releasing devices are protective against ectopic pregnancy

—Another form of contraception is advised in a woman who has previously had an ectopic pregnancy.
* *Expulsion* is most likely during the first month.
  —About 50% of all expulsions take place within 3 months of insertion; after the first year very few are expelled.
  —Among the associated factors are the skill and experience of the person fitting the device; use of an inappropriate size or type of IUD; use in young nulliparous women.
* *Uterine perforation* occurs in about 1/1000 insertions.
  —Most devices can be removed from the peritoneal cavity by laparoscopy but laparotomy is sometimes necessary.
  —Cu-bearing devices tend to form omental masses and adhesions, and should be removed promptly.
* *Pelvic infection*—the risk is increased × 2 but only for the first few weeks after insertion.
  —The major risk factor is the number of sexual partners of the woman and her partner. Monogamous women using a copper device have no increased risk.
* *Lost threads* may be due to unrecognised expulsion; perforation of the uterus (see above); or a normally-sited device with the threads above the external os.
  —The site of the IUD can be checked by ultrasound
  —Threads may be retrieved using a thread retrieval device.

Pregnancy with an IUD in place
* The risk of miscarriage is increased × 5 particularly if the IUD is left in situ: a major associated complication is second-trimester septic abortion.
* Intrauterine candidal infection resulting in fetal death can rarely occur.
* The device should therefore be removed if the threads are accessible: if threads are not visible, counsel about risk of miscarriage and later intrauterine infection.
* Exclude ectopic pregnancy.

CONTRAINDICATIONS

Table 18.2 lists contraindications for parous/nulliparous women.

Table 18.2   Contraindications to the use of an IUD

Contraindication	Nulliparous women	Parous women
Pregnancy	absolute	absolute
Serious pregnancy-related pelvic infection within previous year	absolute	absolute
Active pelvic inflammatory disease	absolute	absolute
Significant congenital uterine anomaly	absolute	absolute
Undiagnosed uterine bleeding	absolute	absolute
Carcinoma of cervix or endometrium	absolute	absolute
Previous ectopic pregnancy	absolute	relative
Risk from bacteraemia, e.g. valvular heart disease, renal dialysis or transplant, or immunosuppressive drugs	absolute	absolute
Multiple sexual partners	relative	relative
Past history of STD	absolute	relative
Menorrhagia	relative	relative
Copper allergy or Wilson's disease	avoid Cu-bearing devices	

BARRIER CONTRACEPTION

- Barrier contraceptives prevent live sperm from entering the cervical canal either by mechanical occlusion (caps and condoms) or by killing sperm (spermicides).
- Condoms are the most popular.
- Caps include vaginal diaphragms, cervical caps, vault caps and vimules (see Further Reading).
- The most commonly used is the diaphragm, which should be:
  —used in conjunction with spermicides
  —fitted before intercourse and removed 6 hours afterwards.
- The use-effectiveness of these methods varies widely depending on the motivation of the couple, but the theoretical effectiveness of caps and condoms is high, with pregnancy rates as low as 2/100 w.y.
- Barrier methods have assumed great importance in the battle against the spread of HIV infection (see p. 110). They should therefore be discussed with ALL couples seeking contraceptive advice, even if they are using another method in addition.

SAFE-PERIOD METHODS

Several methods may be used to detect the fertile and infertile phases in the cycle.

Rhythm method
The lengths of the previous 12 cycles are recorded and the time during which intercourse is to be avoided is between 18 and 11 days before the next period is due to begin. This method is not applicable if the cycle is very irregular, or after recent pregnancy, and may be affected by illness or emotional upset.

Cyclical temperature changes
These can be used in two main ways:
- the couple abstain from sexual intercourse until 3 days after the temperature has risen
- intercourse can take place in the early follicular phase, and time of abstinence is determined by use of the calendar and timing of the temperature rise.

Cervical mucus
- Cervical mucus becomes profuse and watery with a good spinnbarkeit at ovulation.
- The popular 'sympto-thermal' method combines observation of cyclical temperature and cervical mucus changes.

These methods are effective when used consistently by highly-motivated couples, but even then it is reported that accidental pregnancy may occur in up to 14% of women using the 'sympto-thermal' method for 2 years.

COITUS INTERRUPTUS

Male withdrawal is the oldest and most widely used method of contraception. It is simple, moderately effective and without serious side-effects (excluding pregnancy).

MALE AND FEMALE STERILISATION

- Sterilisation in either partner is increasingly popular for birth control. The peak age in women is between 30 and 34 years. The popularity of this irreversible approach is due to the limitations of other, reversible, methods.
- In counselling couples requesting sterilisation the following general points must be borne in mind:
  —The operation (either male or female) must be deemed to be irreversible
  —Alternative methods must have been considered fully
  —Sterilisation of either partner will not stabilise an insecure marriage
  —Agreement to sterilisation must *never* be a prior condition for agreement to undertake termination of pregnancy
  —Childbirth or abortion are stressful times and extra care must be taken to ensure that sterilisation at these times is appropriate

—The small failure rate of all approaches must be explained and that discussion recorded in the casenotes

—If postpartum sterilisation is being requested the couple may be advised to defer operation for some time if the child is sickly at birth

—Written consent must be obtained from the person undergoing the operation, and that of the partner is advisable.

FEMALE STERILISATION

- The current techniques in order of popularity are:
  —*laparoscopy*—the fallopian tubes are occluded by clips or bands or, less commonly now, bipolar diathermy. Unipolar diathermy has a higher level of morbidity including intra-abdominal burns and should therefore be avoided. There is no need to stop oral contraception beforehand
  —*mini-laparotomy*—can be used in women not suitable for laparosocopy: access to the tubes can be, for example, via a proctoscope inserted through a small suprapubic incision
  —*posterior colpotomy*—the tubes are approached through a small incision in the pouch of Douglas; complication rates are higher than for above methods
  —*hysteroscopic techniques* (e.g. diathermy or tubal plugs) require further development.
- The failure rate is between 0.2 and 1% depending on the type of operation and experience of the operator.
- Pregnancy can result from:
  —true method failure
  —surgical error—e.g. misidentification of tubes
  —woman in luteal phase and pregnant at time of operation.
- *Technical failure* is associated with obesity; history of pelvic inflammatory disease; previous abdominal or pelvic surgery; and the skill/experience of the operator.
- *Reversibility*: tubal re-anastomosis will restore fertility in 50–70% of women (depending on the method of sterilisation and the experience of the operator).
  —Ectopic pregnancy can be expected in about 8% of conceptions.

MALE STERILISATION (VASECTOMY)

- This can be performed as an outpatient procedure under local anaesthetic.
- The *vas deferens* is approached through small bilateral scrotal incisions, cut and ligated or diathermied.
- Two sperm-free specimens at 3 and 4 months post operation should be obtained before the patient can be deemed to be sterile.
- The failure rate is 1–4/1000 procedures.

- *Reversibility*: if the technique used for vasectomy is amenable to reversal, sperm will return to the ejaculate in 70–90% of men, and about 30% of their partners will become pregnant.

FURTHER READING

Filshie M, Guillebaud J 1990 Contraception: science and practice. Butterworths, London

Guerts T B P, Goorissen E M, Sitsen J M A 1993 Summary of drug interactions with oral contraceptives. Parthenon Publishing Group, Carnforth

Guillebaud J 1995 Advising women on which pill to take. British Medical Journal 311:1111–1112

Loudon N, Glossier A, Gebbie A 1995 Handbook of family planning, 3rd edn. Churchill Livingstone, Edinburgh

McEwan J 1985 Hormonal methods of contraception and their adverse effect. In: Studd J (ed) Progress in obstetrics and gynaecology 5:259. Churchill Livingstone, Edinburgh

MacRae K, Kay C 1995 Third generation oral contraceptive pills. British Medical Journal 311:1112

THRIFT Consensus Group 1992 Risk of and prophylaxis for venous thromboembolism in hospital patients. British Medical Journal 305:567–574

19. Pelvic infections

PELVIC INFLAMMATORY DISEASE (PID)

Primary An infection which ascends from the lower genital tract due to:

- sexually transmitted diseases (STDs) caused by organisms such as *Chlamydia trachomatis* and *Neisseria gonorrhoeae*. PID is the most common serious complication of STDs, and these organisms cause at least 70% of all cases
  - —Up to 60% of women with gonorrhoea are asymptomatic for months or even years and up to 10% of men may be symptomless carriers
  - —Chlamydial antibodies can be found in up to 70% of women infertile because of tubal damage
  - —There is no history of clinically recognised PID in 30–80% of infertile women with blocked tubes.
- *escherichia coli* and other gut organisms
- replacement of normal vaginal flora (primarily lactobacilli) with organisms associated with 'bacterial vaginosis' (see p. 000), e.g. bacteroides spp., anaerobes, *Mycoplasma hominis* and *Ureaplasma urealyticum*
- iatrogenic—about 15% of all cases: due, for example, to D & C, HSG, termination of pregnancy (TOP) (0.5% post TOP), insertion of an IUD
- after delivery or miscarriage.

Secondary Less than 1% of all cases.

- An infection caused by direct spread from nearby pelvic organs (most often the appendix) *or* other diseases (e.g. schistosomiasis or filariasis).
- A minority of women with PID are HIV positive.

PREVALENCE AND RISK MARKERS

- Pelvic inflammatory disease is rare in women who are not sexually active.
- The overall incidence is 10–13/1000 women of reproductive age, with a peak of 20/1000 in the 15–24 age group.
- Risk markers include:
  - —young age (see above)
  - —multiple sexual partners
  - —use of IUD: (barrier methods and COC protect—see p. 217)
  - —smoking
  - —vaginal douching?

Clinical features of acute PID
- Lower abdominal pain (usually bilateral) is the commonest presenting symptom, which may be accompanied by:
  —abnormal vaginal discharge —nausea and/or vomiting
  —irregular vaginal bleeding —fever
  —dysuria —general malaise.
  —dyspareunia
- Diagnostic accuracy using the above criteria is 35–65%. They can be present in up to 20% of women with no pelvic pathology.
- Among the conditions most frequently causing false-positive or false-negative errors in differential diagnosis are:
  —acute appendicitis —corpus luteum haemorrhage
  —endometriosis —ovarian cysts
  —ectopic pregnancy —inflammatory conditions of
  other organs.
- Lower abdominal and adnexal tenderness, and pain on moving the cervix ('cervical excitation') are found in >90% of women with proven PID.

Diagnosis
- Consider PID in any woman of reproductive age with acute pelvic pain.
- Send endocervical (not high vaginal!) swabs for *C. trachomatis* and *N. gonorrhoeae*.
- Laparoscopy is the gold standard for diagnosis. For positive diagnosis all of the following features must be present:
  —erythema of fallopian tubes
  —oedema and swelling of tubes
  —seropurulent exudate on the surface of the tube from the fimbriated end.
- The inflammation is usually but not invariably bilateral.
- The degrees of severity are:
  —*mild* if these criteria are present but the tubes are mobile and patent
  —*moderate* if the findings are more florid, the tubes are not mobile and their patency is uncertain
  —*severe* if a tubo-ovarian mass or masses are present.
- Swabs can be taken for culture at laparoscopy from the fallopian tubes or the pouch of Douglas: peritoneal fluid can also be cultured.

TREATMENT OF ACUTE PID
- Most women can be treated as outpatients. Among those for whom in-patient treatment may be necessary are the following:
  —failure to respond to or tolerate treatment as outpatient: patient cannot or will not attend for clinical follow-up within 72 hours

—severe disease
—suspected pelvic abscess
—woman is HIV positive
—patient is adolescent (because of importance of adequate therapy to reduce chances of long-term sequelae)
—patient is pregnant
—uncertain diagnosis or other cause of 'acute abdomen' cannot be excluded.

Antibiotic therapy

- Treatment with single agents such as penicillins or tetracyclines is inadequate: cephalosporins do not deal with chlamydia.
- A multiple regimen is required to cover gonococci, chlamydia, Gram-negative organisms and anaerobes. Table 19.1 gives regimens suggested by the Centers for Disease Control and Prevention (CDC) in the USA. For details of dosage, see BNF or Further Reading.

Table 19.1   Antibiotic regimens for acute PID. Source: CDC, Atlanta

In-patient	Regimen 1	Regimen 2
	Cefoxitin i.v. plus doxycycline i.v. or orally. Continue for at least 48 hrs after clinical condition is significantly improved, then give oral doxycycline for a total of 14 days	Clindamycin i.v. plus gentamicin i.v. or i.m. Then as for regimen 1 with oral clindamycin as an alternative to doxycycline
Outpatient	Regimen 1	Regimen 2
	Cefoxitin i.m. (plus probenecid) or other third-generation cephalosporin and oral doxycycline for 14 days	Oral ofloxacin plus clindamycin or metronidazole for 14 days

Surgery

The main role of surgery in the management of acute PID is after rupture of a tubo-ovarian abscess and to drain a pyosalpinx.

Contact tracing

Male partners should be examined for STDs.

Sequelae

- *Chronic pelvic pain*—will follow in 20% of affected women. Of these 60–70% will be infertile and/or have dyspareunia.
- *Subfertility* due to tubal damage and occlusion. It occurs in:
  —10% of women after a single episode of PID
  —20% after two episodes
  —40% after three or more episodes.

- *Ectopic pregnancy*—PID increases the risk × 7–10.
- *Recurrent PID*—the patient classically complains of:
  —heavy and irregular menses
  —dysmenorrhoea
  —dyspareunia
  —chronic pelvic pain
  —infertility.

There may also be chronic vaginal discharge. The uterus and adnexae are tender; the former is often fixed in retroversion. The condition which most closely mimics chronic PID is endometriosis.

FURTHER READING

Centers for Disease Control and Prevention 1991 Pelvic inflammatory disease: guidelines for prevention and management. Morbidity and Mortality Weekly Report 40 (RR-5):1–25. CDC, Atlanta
Tindall V R 1990 Jeffcoate's principles of gynaecology, 5th edn. Butterworths, London

20. Disorders of micturition

URINARY INCONTINENCE

20–30% of women over the age of 65 years are said to suffer from a significant degree of urinary incontinence.

Definitions
- *Stress incontinence* is the involuntary loss of a small amount of urine during exercise, coughing, sneezing, etc. It occurs when the intravesical pressure exceeds the maximum urethral pressure (in the absence of detrusor activity).
- *Urge incontinence* is the involuntary loss of urine associated with a strong desire to micturate.
  —*Motor urgency* is associated with uninhibited detrusor contractions
  —*Sensory urgency* is due to irritative lesions (e.g. cystitis, calculus, tumour) in which the detrusor is stable.
- *Reflex incontinence* is the involuntary loss of urine due to abnormal spinal reflex activity in the absence of the sensation to micturate.
- *Overflow incontinence* is the involuntary loss of urine when the intravesical pressure exceeds maximum urethral pressure due to bladder distension and in the absence of detrusor activity.
- *True incontinence* is the involuntary loss of urine due to a defect in the anatomical integrity of the urinary tract.

INVESTIGATION

Past history
- Past medical and surgical history, e.g. STD; polio; surgery to spine or genitourinary tract; cerebrovascular accident; cerebral, spinal or pelvic trauma
- Gynaecological and obstetric history—particularly of rapid or slow labours, 'difficult' delivery (especially with forceps) or large infants
- Previous urological complaints (e.g. enuresis, urinary infections, haematuria)
- Family history (e.g. enuresis, diabetes)
- Concurrent disease (e.g. multiple sclerosis, Parkinson's disease).

Present complaint
- *Stress*—leakage with e.g. coughing, sneezing, exercise or sexual intercourse?

- *Irritative*—frequency or urgency of micturition; urge incontinence; nocturia?
- *Voiding*—hesitancy; intermittency of flow; incomplete bladder emptying?
- *Quantity of leakage*—dribbles; flooding; clothes soaked; number of pads used?
- *Social implications*—perceived effect on partner and friends; effect on sexual relations, exercise or going to social events?

Symptomatic guide to detrusor activity
- It is very difficult to differentiate genuine stress incontinence (GSI) from detrusor instability (DI) symptomatically. In women with symptoms suggesting GSI, urodynamic tests will demonstrate DI in 10–15% of cases.
- The information box gives some guide to the stability of the detrusor.

Guide to detrusor stability	
Stable	*Unstable*
• Only symptom is stress incontinence	• Urgency and urge incontinence
• Micturition normal	• Frequency and nocturia
• Urine loss small	• Urine loss great

Pelvic examination
The purpose is to:
- demonstrate incontinence and/or utero-vaginal prolapse
- detect any other pelvic pathology
- note other features such as oestrogenisation of the vaginal wall, the ability to contract the pelvic floor and scarring from any previous surgery.

Urine microscopy and culture are compulsory. *Cytology* should be performed if haematuria, sensory urgency or bladder pain are present.

Frequency and volume chart
Urodynamic tests are necessary because 'the bladder is a bad witness' (see above).
- Tests of urine flow will differentiate abnormal from normal voiding and can evaluate the results of surgical treatment of the bladder neck.
- *Cystometry* primarily tests the reservoir function of the bladder. *Filling cystometrogram (CMG)* assesses detrusor activity and leakage during the filling phase. *Voiding CMG* assesses urinary

flow and will differentiate obstruction from an underactive bladder if detrusor pressure is measured simultaneously.

- *Urethral pressure profile* assesses urethral closure pressure.
- *Video-cystourethrography* combines assessment of the anatomical relationship of the urethra, urethro-vesical junction and bladder base with measurement of bladder pressure, urine flow and volume. It is especially suitable for the assessment of complex cases, e.g. failed surgery.

Among the indications for urodynamic investigations are:
—anyone being considered for surgery because of the presence of DI in 10–15% of women whose symptoms and signs suggest GSI
—irritative symptoms which do not respond to treatment
—all complicated cases, e.g. women with neuropathy or suspected obstruction.

An *intravenous urogram* will help to exclude congenital anomalies, calculi or ureteric fistulae.

Cystoscopy should be carried out if there is sensory urgency with a small-capacity bladder to exclude interstitial cystitis or malignancy.

GENUINE STRESS INCONTINENCE (GSI)

Aetiology
- Continence in the female is achieved because the urethro-vesical junction and proximal urethra lie above the pelvic floor muscles and are, therefore, intra-abdominal structures.
- Any rise in intra-abdominal pressure is transmitted equally to the bladder and proximal urethra which preserves the pressure gradient and maintains the positive urethral closure pressure (see section (a), Fig. 20.1).
- GSI will tend to occur when an alteration in position of the bladder neck in relation to the pelvic flow (section (b), Fig. 20.1) means that most of the urethra is below it.
- Any increase in intra-abdominal pressure will increase intravesical but not urethral pressure. The former will exceed the latter (i.e. there is a negative urethral closure pressure) and a small amount of urine will be lost.
- These changes may or may not be accompanied by a cystocele.
- Other features found in association with stress incontinence are funnelling of the bladder neck on exertion or straining (without detrusor activity) and a short functional length of the urethra.
- Among the possible causative factors are:
  —childbirth—vaginal deliveries in particular
  —pelvic surgery
  —menopause
  —pelvic pathology, e.g. utero-vaginal prolapse; pelvic masses

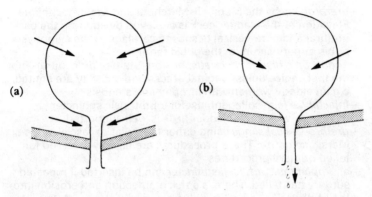

Fig 20.1 Stress incontinence. (a) Rise in intra-abdominal pressure preserves pressure gradient. (b) Genuine stress incontinence: alteration in position of bladder neck to pelvic flow.

—congenital—connective tissue abnormalities; very short urethra; female 'epispadias'.

TREATMENT OF GSI

- *Physiotherapy*
  —Pelvic floor exercises are useful prophylaxis after childbirth.
  —Up to 60% of women can be helped by conscientious use of, for example, vaginal cones.
  —Electrical stimulation of pelvic muscles.
- *Drug therapy*
  —Genuine stress incontinence is not amenable to treatment with anticholinergic drugs but adrenergic drugs may help.
  —Correction of oestrogen deficiency in postmenopausal women may be beneficial.
- *Surgery* aims to achieve some or all of the following effects:
  —restoration of the position of the proximal urethra as an intra-abdominal structure
  —increase in the urethral closure pressure
  —increase in functional urethral length
  —increase in support to bladder neck and therefore its competence.
- *Anterior colporrhaphy* treats anterior vaginal wall prolapse but is less likely to cure stress incontinence.
- *Primary suprapubic procedures* are reported to have success rates of 80–90%. Among them are:
  —*colposuspension* by the Burch technique in which the bladder neck and anterior vaginal wall are elevated by suturing the para-vaginal fascia to the ipsilateral ileo-pectineal ligament

—*urethropexy* by the Marshall–Marchetti and Krantz technique. Elevation of the bladder neck is achieved by suturing the para-urethral and para-vesical tissues to cartilage of the symphysis pubis or periosteum of the pubic ramus

—*endoscopic bladder neck suspension* (Stamey procedure)—not the first choice unless vaginal access and capacity are limited, e.g. in elderly women with atrophy and stenosis

—*injectables* (e.g. collagen), useful for intrinsic sphincter deficiency where the bladder neck is well supported

—*urethro-vesical slings* using either muscular or fascial strips or Mersilene gauze. These procedures are usually reserved for failed primary procedures

—an *implantable artificial sphincter* can be inserted if repeated surgery has failed. There is a risk of infection and erosion into the urethra

—*urinary diversion procedures* may ultimately be necessary in a few patients in whom all other methods have failed. The construction of an ileal conduit is the usual method.

DETRUSOR INSTABILITY (DI)

Aetiology

The cause of primary instability of the detrusor remains unknown. It may be a variant of normal bladder function because:

- it is the natural state in all infants
- about 10% of the population never develop stable bladder function
- urodynamic studies suggest that it may be present in 60–70% of 'normal' women.

It may rarely be secondary to an upper motor neurone lesion, e.g. multiple sclerosis leading to detrusor hyperreflexia.

TREATMENT OF DI

In general, treatment of primary DI is unsatisfactory.

- *Bladder training* is a simple approach with as good or better results than any other remedy. It can be used in conjunction with drug therapy.
- *Drug therapy.* Drugs with anticholinergic activity may be beneficial, usually only for as long as they are taken. Oxybutaline may be effective intravesically in refractory cases.
- *Surgery* is not routinely indicated. Such radical procedures as clam cystoplasty or detrusor myomectomy may be rarely indicated for refractory idiopathic or hyperreflexic DI.

GENITOURINARY FISTULAE

- *Uretero-vaginal fistulae* usually follow hysterectomy (particularly radical surgery).

- *High vesico-vaginal fistulae* can follow lower segment caesarean section, uterine rupture, hysterectomy or radiotherapy for cervical carcinoma. The ureteric orifices may be near the edge.
- *Mid-vaginal vesico-vaginal fistulae* may be caused by pressure necrosis after prolonged obstructed labour or colporrhaphy fistulae. These are the commonest and are mostly due either to pressure necrosis or trauma by rotational forceps.
- *Urethral fistulae* may occasionally be so large as to virtually destroy the whole urethra and the bladder neck.

MANAGEMENT

Some defects will close spontaneously and all will heal to some extent if given enough time. Even if spontaneous closure does not occur, surgery should be deferred to allow maximum tissue healing. If secondary to radiation this may take up to a year or more.

Pre-operative management
- In addition to attending to the patient's general health, among the pre-operative investigations which should be carried out are urine culture and sensitivity, intravenous urography, cystoscopy and assessment under anaesthesia.
- If the fistula is associated with radiotherapy for neoplasm a biopsy of the edge should be taken to exclude residual tumour activity.

Operative closure
Technical details of closure are found in Further Reading, but these are among the important points.
- All but the simplest cases should be referred to centres or surgeons with special expertise.
- Most urethro-vaginal and vesico-vaginal fistulae can be repaired vaginally by dissection and repair in layers.
- The bladder wall closure must be watertight.
- Over 70% of fistulae can be closed at the first attempt, falling to about 30% if three or more repairs have previously been attempted.
- Continuous catheter drainage is necessary for a minimum of 10 days (up to 3 weeks for radiation fistulae). The drainage system should be closed.
- In any subsequent pregnancy all deliveries should be by elective caesarean section.

VOIDING DIFFICULTIES

THE URETHRAL SYNDROME

Definition
- Recurrent attacks of frequent and painful micturition not associated with any significant abnormality in the urinary tract and irrespective of the presence or absence of bacteriuria.
- Used synonymously with 'recurrent cystitis'.

AETIOLOGY

- *Infective*—significant bacteriuria ($>10^6$ organisms/ml) is present in only about half of the cases. The commonest infective agents are normal bowel flora. Among the others are *T. vaginalis, N. gonorrhoeae* and *C. trachomatis*. Tuberculosis of the bladder is a rare cause.
- *Gynaecological*—e.g. postmenopausal oestrogen deficiency.
- *Chemical or allergic reactions*—may be due to soaps, douches, deodorants, contraceptive foam or anti-oxidants in condoms. It can also arise by wearing nylon underwear or tights.
- *Sexual*—its occasional association with first intercourse has led to the term 'honeymoon cystitis'.
- *Psychological*—anxiety and neuroticism are not infrequent associations. Which is cause and which effect is not always entirely clear.
- *Bladder problems*—DI is present in over 25% of cases. A bladder tumour is a rare cause but it must be suspected if there is haematuria.
- *Other causes*. Multiple sclerosis may rarely present in this fashion.

MANAGEMENT

- A full history is vital. Haematuria requires full investigation. A full gynaecological assessment is essential.
- Routinely test urine for protein, glucose, blood and infection.
- An optimistic attitude and positive approach to treatment is important because there is often an understandably large functional overlay in these patients.
- Simple remedies may be the most effective, e.g. perineal and introital hygiene: potassium citrate and sodium bicarbonate with a high fluid intake.
- Start antibiotic therapy if symptoms do not subside within 48 hours of commencing a high fluid intake.
- Try hormone replacement therapy in menopausal women.

FURTHER READING

Royal College of Physicians 1995 Incontinence—cause, management and provision of services. RCP, London

Shaw R W, Soutter W P, Stanton S L (eds) 1996 Gynaecology, 2nd edn. Churchill Livingstone, Edinburgh

Tindall V R 1990 Jeffcoate's Principles of Gynaecology, 5th edn. Butterworths, London

21. Uterine displacement and utero-vaginal prolapse

RETROVERSION

- Mobile retroversion of the uterus is a variant of normal occurring in over 25% of women.
- It is usually asymptomatic and too many gynaecological symptoms have been attributed to it in the past. Backache is more frequently due to other conditions.
- An associated positioning of the ovaries in the pouch of Douglas may be a cause of dyspareunia.
- Retroversion is not a cause of subfertility.
- An acutely retroverted gravid uterus may become 'impacted' in the pelvis as the uterus enlarges. Acute retention of urine may result.
- Mobile retroversion can be temporarily corrected by insertion of a Hodge pessary into the vagina.
- Fixed retroversion is most frequently due to pelvic inflammatory disease (p. 231) or endometriosis (p. 197). The associated symptoms and signs and the management depend on the underlying disease.
- The traditional remedy of 'ventrosuspension' by laparoscopy or laparotomy to shorten the round ligaments by suturing them to the rectus sheath cannot be justified.

UTERO-VAGINAL PROLAPSE

Support of the pelvic floor
- The uterus and vagina are mainly supported by the *levatores ani* muscles of the pelvic floor which form a downwards and forwards sloping gutter slung around the midline structures.
- The three components of the *levatores ani* are *ischio-coccygeus, ilio-coccygeus, and pubo-coccygeus*.

Definition of prolapse
The downward displacement of the uterus and/or vagina towards or through the introitus. The bladder, urethra, rectum and bowel may be secondarily involved.
Prolapse has three degrees of severity:
- first degree: descent of the cervix, to the introitus
- second degree: descent of the cervix, but not the whole uterus, through the introitus

- third degree (procidentia): descent of the cervix and the whole uterus through the introitus.

AETIOLOGY

Attenuation of the support mechanisms may occur as a result of:
- childbirth—prolapse is uncommon in nulliparous women. Prolonged labours with difficult vaginal deliveries may predispose to the development of prolapse subsequently. Precipitate labour may indicate some degree of deficiency of the pelvic floor which may later express itself as prolapse
- postmenopausal atrophy
- chronic elevation of intra-abdominal pressure due, for example, to obesity or a chronic cough.

VAGINAL WALL PROLAPSE

- A prolapse of the lowest third of the anterior vaginal wall involves the urethra and is therefore termed a *urethrocele*.
- In the upper two thirds the bladder is involved and it is, therefore, a *cystocele*.
- A prolapse of the pouch of Douglas is an *enterocele* because the hernial sac contains gut or omentum.
- A prolapse of the posterior vaginal wall brings the rectum with it and is therefore a *rectocele*. (This is not to be confused with prolapse of the rectal mucosa through the anus.)

Symptoms and signs
- The commonest symptoms are:
  —a feeling of 'something coming down'
  —awareness of a lump protruding from the vulva
  —discomfort and backache
  —possible stress incontinence because the urethra lies caudal to the pelvic floor (see p. 237) and not primarily because of loss of the posterior urethro-vesical angle
  —urinary retention or difficulty with defecation occur occasionally in severe vaginal wall prolapse.
- Examination is best carried out with the patient in the left lateral position using a Sims speculum.
- A volsellum may be applied to the cervix so that traction will demonstrate the severity of uterine prolapse. This can cause marked discomfort and should be performed gently.

MANAGEMENT
Prevention
- Avoidance of perineal overstretching during labour and adequate repair thereafter
- Encouragement to persist with postnatal pelvic floor exercises

- Avoidance of obesity and cigarette smoking
- Appropriate use of hormone replacement therapy in some postmenopausal women.

TREATMENT

In established cases the appropriate treatment will be determined by the following features:
- the severity of symptoms
- the extent of the signs—asymptomatic first-degree prolapse does not require treatment
- age, parity and wish for further pregnancies
- the patient's sexual activity
- the presence of aggravating features, e.g. *the results of treatment will be poor unless the obese patient loses weight and the smoker stops smoking*
- urinary symptoms (see p. 237)
- other gynaecological problems, e.g. menorrhagia.

Conservative treatment
- Pelvic floor exercises will improve the tone of the pelvic floor muscles in the young parous woman but they will not produce much benefit for the woman with significant utero-vaginal prolapse.
- Ring pessaries may be used temporarily during or after pregnancy. They can be used for longer-term control in the woman who refuses or is unfit for surgery.

Surgical treatment
- Prolapse is not a life-threatening condition but surgery has its morbidity and occasional mortality.
- *Anterior colporrhaphy* is appropriate for the repair of a cystocele. It is less likely to be effective in the correction of genuine stress incontinence (see p. 236).
- *Posterior colpoperineorrhaphy* will control a rectocele but an enterocele will have to be dealt with separately.
- *Manchester (Fothergill) repair* may still be appropriate for all degrees of prolapse in experienced hands.
  —It combines shortening of the transverse cervical ligament with amputation of the cervix and anterior colporrhaphy.
  —It may not deal adequately with an enterocele.
  —It is appropriate for the small number of women with severe prolapse who wish to have further children.
  —Full amputation of the cervix may not be necessary in less severe cases; removal of an anterior wedge of cervix may be adequate.
  —Caesarean section is necessary in any subsequent pregnancy.
- *Vaginal hysterectomy* is now the standard operation for utero-vaginal prolapse even in the absence of uterine pathology as

long as the uterus is not enlarged to a size greater than the
equivalent of a 12-week pregnancy.
- It is also the operation of choice:
  —if an enterocele is present (the utero-sacral ligaments can be
   used to obliterate the hernial sac)
  —for a procidentia
  —if the uterus is atrophic.

FURTHER READING

Shaw R W, Soutter W P, Stanton S L (eds) 1996 Gynaecology, 2nd edn. Churchill
    Livingstone, Edinburgh
Tindall V R 1990 Jeffcoate's principles of gynaecology, 5th edn. Butterworths, London

22. Intersexes and congenital malformations of the genital tract

INTERSEX

- An intersex is an individual in whom there is discordance between chromosomal, gonadal, internal genital and phenotypic sex or the sex of rearing.
- This may declare itself:
  —at birth because of ambiguous external genitalia
  —during childhood because of precocious puberty
  —during adolescence because pubertal changes are inappropriate to presumed gender or because puberty fails to occur.
- Some types of intersexuality may never become apparent, e.g. the XYY male or XXX female.

CLASSIFICATION OF INTERSEXES

Chromosomal abnormalities
- *Turner's syndrome*—see page 39
- *Triple X female.* Some may have oligomenorrhoea and/or premature menopause but others go undetected
- *Klinefelter's syndrome (47 XXY).* Characterised by azoospermia, hypoplasia of seminiferous tubules, and perhaps gynaecomastia and eunuchoidism
- *Aberration of H-Y antigen*
  —XX male—maleness is due to translocation of the H-Y antigens onto an autosome or one of the X chromosomes
  —XY female—due to functional absence of H-Y. The clinical features are variable.

Gonadal aberrations
- *True hermaphrodite* – both testicular and ovarian tissue is present. External and internal genital sex vary widely. The commonest chromosomal structure is 46 XX
- *Gonadal agenesis*—there is no gonadal tissue but no other congenital abnormality. The phenotype is female and the karyotype can be either 46 XX or 46 XY
- *Absent anti-Müllerian factor*—noticeable at birth because of dubious genitalia. A normal vagina, uterus and tubes are present but with bilateral testes. The karyotype is 46 XY. The testis can produce androgen but not anti-Müllerian factor.

End-organ resistance
- *Testicular feminisation*—see page 184
- *Varying degree of hypospadias*—these may be due to relative cytosol receptor deficiency
- Familial or sporadic *5α-reductase deficiency* will also result in the birth of children with dubious genitalia but who are genetically male. Virilisation occurs at puberty.

Female intersexuality
This may be due to:
- *Congenital adrenal hyperplasia (CAH)*—the commonest cause of intersex.
  - —It is most frequently caused by a deficiency of 21-hydroxylase and therefore insufficient cortisol and aldosterone are produced. A female fetus will be exposed to an excess of adrenal androgens and virilisation will result
  - —Profound salt loss can be life-threatening in the neonate.
- *Ingestion of 19-norsteroid progestogens* during pregnancy; or (rarely) excess maternal androgen production. A female fetus is born virilised to a greater or lesser extent.

MANAGEMENT
- Check:
  - —buccal smear karyotype
  - —urinary 17-oxosteroids
  - —urinary pregnanetriol $\Big\}$ increased in CAH
  - —plasma 17α-hydroxyprogesterone
  - —plasma electrolytes.
- Treat salt-losing CAH with glucocorticoids (permanently)
- An X-ray after gastrografin instillation into the urogenital sinus will allow visualisation of the internal genitalia
- In difficult cases assign the sex of rearing to the sex which can be made adequate for coitus.

LATER MANAGEMENT
- Any corrective surgery to the external genitalia is best carried out before the age of 3 years.
- Exploratory laparotomy is sometimes indicated but usually only in male intersexes and in true hermaphroditism.
- A male (XY) intersex showing virilism at birth will probably virilise at puberty. If the assigned sex is female the testes will need to be removed before virilisation begins at puberty.
- XY gonads should be removed in gonadal dysgenesis because of the 25% risk of malignancy.
- Testes should probably also be removed after puberty in testicular feminisation because of slightly increased risk of seminoma formation.

- If an artificial vagina is required it is best to wait until physical growth is complete.
- In gonadal agenesis or after removal of gonads, oestrogens will be required to produce secondary sex characteristics at the appropriate time. Cyclical oestrogens and progestogens should be used if a uterus is present because of the risk of endometrial carcinoma if unopposed oestrogens are given over a long period of time.

CONGENITAL MALFORMATIONS OF THE GENITAL TRACT

Among the congenital anomalies which can occur are:
- *fusion of the labia* (rare)
- *complete absence or duplication of the vulva* (both rare)
- *persistence of the cloaca*—a serious problem. Urinary and faecal incontinence result
- *defects of the posterior cloacal wall*—faecal continence is maintained by pelvic floor muscles
- *defects in anterior cloacal wall*—affect urinary and genital tracts. Minor abnormalities do not cause undue problems but major defects can result in bladder extrophy and deficient anterior abdominal wall
- *ectopic ureter*—usually an accessory ureter. The site of the orifice in relation to the bladder sphincter mechanism determines whether incontinence is present or not. The orifice can be difficult to locate and may not show up on excretion urography
- *septate vagina*—not uncommon and only requires division if it poses mechanical problems for coitus or childbirth. May accompany a uterine anomaly
- *transverse vaginal membrane* (including imperforate hymen). Will result in haematocolpos and cryptomenorrhoea (see p. 183)
- *incomplete or absent vagina*—both are usually associated with absence of the uterus (and possible renal tract anomalies). Construction of an artificial vagina may have to be considered if the vagina is non-existent. Vulvo-vaginoplasty is a relatively simple and effective procedure (see Further Reading).

UTERINE ANOMALIES

- Agenesis or arrested development of one Müllerian duct will result in one of the following (see Fig. 22.1):
  (i) unicornuate uterus (with tube)
  (ii) unicornuate uterus plus some form of rudimentary horn
  (iii) the rudimentary horn may not be joined to the unicornuate uterus.

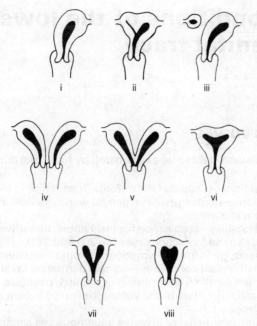

Fig 22.1   Congenital malformations of the genital tract

- Failure of, or incomplete, fusion of Müllerian duct may produce the following:
  - (iv)   double uterus (didelphys) with septate vagina
  - (v)   double uterus (didelphys) with normal vagina
  - (vi)   arcuate deformity
  - (vii, viii) septate or sub-septate uterus.
- These anomalies may be associated with dysmenorrhoea, dyspareunia, miscarriage, pre-term labour, intrauterine growth retardation or fetal malpresentation.
- Surgical correction is only indicated for the more severe anomalies which have already produced problems.
- A uterine septum can be removed hysteroscopically.

FURTHER READING

Shaw R W, Soutter W P, Stanton S L (eds) 1996 Gynaecology, 2nd edn. Churchill Livingstone, Edinburgh

Tindall V R 1990 Jeffcoate's principles of gynaecology, 5th edn. Butterworths, London

23. Conditions of the lower genital tract

PRURITUS VULVAE

Some local causes—all can be exacerbated by heat, moisture and friction.
- Fungal infections—*Candida* (see p. 259), *Tinea cruris*
- Viral infections—herpes genitalis, genital warts, molluscum contagiosum (poxvirus)
- Parastic infestation—scabies, pediculosis pubis, threadworms
- Sexually transmitted infections (see pp. 260 and 261) trichomoniasis, gonorrhoea, lymphogranuloma venereum
- Local dermatological conditions—contact dermatitis (allergic or irritant), lichen simplex, seborrhoeic dermatitis, psoriasis, etc.
- Non-neoplastic disorders of the vulva (previously known as 'vulval dystrophy')
- Tumours—intraepithelial or invasive squamous cell carcinoma
- Miscellaneous—foreign bodies, poor genital hygiene.

Some generalised causes
- Part of generalised dermatosis
- Part of general medical disorder, e.g. diabetes mellitus, liver disease, thyroid disease, Crohn's disease, chronic renal failure, polycythaemia, chronic lymphatic leukaemia
- Drug reactions
- Psychogenic causes.

SWELLING OF AND AROUND THE VULVA

Among the causes are:
- trauma causing a haematoma
- infections (see above)
- utero-vaginal prolapse (see p. 242)
- cysts—sebaceous, inclusion dermoid, Wolffian duct remnants, endometriosis
- varicose veins
- enlargement of Bartholin's gland
  —*Bartholin's adenitis* The gland is acutely painful and swollen. It is often due to a gonococcal infection but is not infrequently caused by straphylococci, streptococci or Gram-negative bacilli. Any abscess should be incised and drained. After an infection has occurred the main duct of the gland may be

blocked and a Bartholin's cyst will form. Marsupialisation rather than excision is probably the best management but not during acute infection.
—*Tumours* These are rare but may be benign adenomas or carcinoma (adenocarcinoma more than squamous— see p. 254).
- Urethral and para-urethral conditions—urethral prolapse, diverticulum or caruncle, cyst of Skene's para-urethral glands
- Inguinal hernia or hydrocele of Canal of Nuck
- Benign neoplasms: e.g. papilloma, fibroma, lipoma, hidradenoma (tumour of sweat glands)
- Malignant neoplasms: primary—squamous cell carcinoma, melanoma, sarcoma; secondary tumours.

NON-NEOPLASTIC EPITHELIAL DISORDERS OF THE VULVA

- Vulval atrophy is normal in elderly women and is symptomless. No treatment is necessary.
- The term 'non-neoplastic epithelial disorders of skin and mucosa of the vulva' has replaced the term 'vulval dystrophies'. They comprise a group of different conditions characterised by disorders of epithelial growth and maturation.
- The characteristic symptom is pruritus.
- Areas of abnormality can appear red, white or pigmented. They may be raised, warty or flat. The correct diagnosis can often be made clinically after careful consideration of the age of the patient, the appearance of the lesion, the condition of the skin elsewhere. If there is doubt about the diagnosis or suspicion of malignancy, biopsy is mandatory. Those with abnormal and disordered epithelial activity (cellular atypia) are sometimes pre-malignant.

CLASSIFICATION

Lichen sclerosus (formerly hypoplastic dystrophy)
A thinning condition of the vulva which is associated with paradoxically increased cell turnover.
- It is of unknown (possibly auto-immune) aetiology. There is an association with some other auto-immune conditions such as achlorhydria and primary biliary cirrhosis.
- Clinically, there may be dyspareunia or vulval pain in addition to pruritus.
- Although traditionally considered to be benign it can be found adjacent to about 30% of vulval cancers. It may itself progress to cancer in about 3% of cases.
- It mainly occurs in older women but can be found in all age groups.
- The commonest sites are the vulva and perianal area but extra-

genital lesions may develop. It begins with small, irregular, flat-topped, white papules often having a central keratotic plug. The patches become atrophic and coalesce. The skin is paper-thin and may break down. The introitus may shrink causing dyspareunia.
- It involves non-genital skin in 20% of affected women.

Histology
- Atrophic thinning of the epidermis with hyperkeratosis
- Absence of dermal papillae and elastic tissue
- Hyaline replacement of the collagen fibres
- Lymphocytic infiltration of deep layers.

Squamous cell hyperplasia
Formerly hyperplastic dystrophy without atypia. Thickening of the epithelium without identifiable cause and without cellular abnormalities: of low pre-malignant potential.

Other dermatoses
E.g. seborrhoeic dermatitis, psoriasis, lichen planus. Dermatological conditions comprise 60% of cases referred to vulval clinics, highlighting the need for joint gynaecological/dermatological consultations.

Paget's disease
This is a separate pre-malignancy. In some cases it is associated with an underlying adenocarcinoma and can itself become invasive.

VULVAL INTRAEPITHELIAL NEOPLASIA (VIN)

'VIN' replaces previous confusing descriptive terms for hypertrophic dystrophies with varying degrees of cellular atypia. There are two distinct subgroups.
- A group affecting women over 50 years of age who present with discrete lesions not related to wart virus infection. These are potentially malignant lesions with progression occurring in up to 5% of *treated* cases. The majority of these lesions may progess to cancer if neglected.
- A group of younger women presenting with multifocal intraepithelial neoplasia—cervical intraepithelial neoplasia, vaginal intraepithelial neoplasia (VAIN), anal intraepithelial neoplasia (AIN) and VIN—affecting different areas of the lower genital tract. This condition is associated with wart virus or human papillomavirus (HPV) infection and is also associated with sexual promiscuity, smoking and immunosuppression (e.g. in renal transplant patients and users of systemic steroids).

- As with the more common cervical intraepithelial neoplasia (CIN) VIN is graded into three subsets:
  —VIN 1 (mild cellular atypia)
  —VIN 2 (moderate cellular atypia)
  —VIN 3 (severe cellular atypia including carcinoma in situ). In VIN 3 atypical cells occupy the full thickness of the epithelium without any stromal invasion.
- It may present as well-defined reddish-brown, moist, papular or plaque-like lesions accompanied by pruritus. Growth is slow but the lesions tend to coalesce and invasive carcinoma will supervene if the lesion is neglected.

Histology
- Hyperplasia (acanthosis) and irregular thickening of epidermis
- Distorted rete ridges
- Hyperkeratosis
- Chronic inflammatory cell infiltrate.

Leukoplakia is a descriptive term for irregular thickening and whitening of the vulval skin that is seen in several pathological conditions. It should not be used as a diagnostic term.

MANAGEMENT OF NON-NEOPLASTIC EPITHELIAL DISORDERS OF VULVA

Exclude or treat:
- deficiencies of iron, riboflavin, vitamin B_{12} and folic acid
- achlorhydria
- allergies (clothing, cosmetics, toilet preparations)
- generalised dermatoses
- diabetes mellitus
- fungal infections.

Lichen sclerosus
- Patients with typical appearances of lichen sclerosus need not have biopsies but areas in which there is any question of malignancy should have several widely spaced biopsies of vulval skin.
- Severe hyperkeratosis which is causing fissuring of the skin can be softened by 2% salicylic acid ointment.
- Pruritus responds to a short, sharp course of potent fluorinated steroids, e.g. Dermovate applied twice daily for 1–2 months. Once controlled, long-term use of a mild steroid cream with an antifungal, e.g. Trimovate, may be needed.
- Testosterone cream is ineffective.
- Vulvectomy or local excision of lesions should be reserved for those cases in which VIN coexists with higher risk of carcinoma or the patient suffers intractable symptoms. The condition can recur after vulvectomy and even skin grafting of the site. Laser therapy, cryosurgery and topical therapy with 5-fluorouracil have also been suggested.

Vulval intraepithelial neoplasia (VIN)

- The definitive treatment is wide local excision which may require removal of all the vulva in widespread disease.
- Where possible reconstructive plastic surgery should be used (rotational skin flaps or split skin grafts).
- Paget's disease requires wide excision because histological abnormalities spread beyond the edge of the clinically affected areas and recurrence is common.
- The factors to be considered in planning treatment are:
  —the certainty of the diagnosis. On the one hand the lesion may not in fact be neoplastic and on the other there may be areas of invasion which have been overlooked
  —the age of the patient and her sexual activity. The effect of complete vulvectomy on a young woman may be devastating
  —the size and location of the lesion
  —the health of the rest of the vulva, e.g. the presence of infection or chronic epithelial dystrophy
  —the ease of long-term follow-up. Local excision demands follow-up.

INVASIVE TUMOURS OF THE VULVA

- Vulval cancer is a disease of older women. The mean age of affected women is about 60 years, and 75% of cases occur in women aged 50 years or over.
- It forms about 5% of all female genital tract cancers.
- There is an association with nulliparity and cigarette smoking.
- 90% of malignant vulval neoplasms are squamous, and most develop in association with lichen sclerosus and VIN. Chronic granulomatous diseases of the vulva, e.g. syphilis, granuloma inguinale or lymphogranuloma venereum, predispose to vulval cancer.
- Between 15 and 30% of women with vulval cancer have had, or will develop, intraepithelial or invasive lesions of the cervix.

PRESENTATION AND SPREAD OF SQUAMOUS CARCINOMA

- An ulcer or papillary lesion may develop after a period of intractable pruritus.
- Continued growth is ultimately accompanied by bleeding, secondary infection and pain.
- Delayed presentation is a major problem.
- The commonest sites are as follows: labia 70% (labia majora 3 times as common as labia minora); clitoris 15%; perineum or fourchette 5%; remainder 10%.
- Most squamous cell carcinomas of the vulva are well differentiated.
- The primary route of spread is lymphatic (see Fig. 23.1).

—Spread occurs first to the superficial and deep inguinal and femoral nodes, then to the external iliac and obturator nodes.

—The common iliac and para-aortic nodes are involved in late cases.

—Contralateral involvement is not uncommon in tumours near the midline because of the extensive anastomosis of the lymphatic network.

- Local growth progressively involves the urethra, vagina, anus and, occasionally, the bladder or rectum.

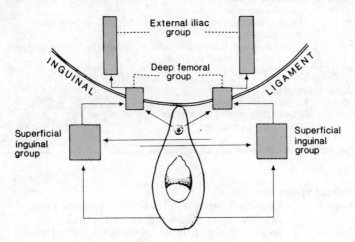

Fig 23.1   Carcinoma of vulva: lymphatic spread

CLINICAL STAGING OF SQUAMOUS CARCINOMA

- Clinical staging is unreliable: palpation of inguinal nodes is not a good guide to involvement; palpable enlarged nodes may not be affected by tumour in up to 40% of cases, and lack of enlargement may mask involvement in a similar number.
- Involvement of nodes is an important prognostic sign, as in other malignant tumours.
- In women with squamous carcinoma the survival rate without node involvement is 75%; with node involvement, 40%.
- Staging can either use a TNM (Tumour, Nodes, Metastasis) classification (see information box) or FIGO clinical staging.

Squamous carcinoma of the vulva: TNM classification

Primary tumour (T):
T1   Tumour confined to the vulva <2 cm in diameter
T2   Tumour confined to the vulva >2 cm in diameter
T3   Tumour of any size with adjacent spread to the urethra and/or vagina, and/or anus
T4   Tumour of any size infiltrating the bladder (including the upper part of the urethra) mucosa, and/or the rectal mucosa and/or fixed to the bone

Regional lymph nodes (N):
N0   No nodes palpable
N1   Nodes palpable in either groin, not enlarged, mobile (not clinically suspicious of neoplasm)
N2   Nodes palpable in either one or both groins, enlarged, firm and mobile (clinically suspicious of neoplasm)
N3   Fixed or ulcerated nodes

Distant metastases (M):
M0   No clinical metastases
M1a   Palpable deep pelvic lymph nodes
M1b   Other distant metastases.

Clinical stage groups

Stage I   Lesions 2 cm or less confined to the vulva or perineum. No lymph node metastases
Stage Ia   As above with stromal invasion no greater than 1 mm
Stage Ib   Stromal invasion >1 mm
Stage II   Lesions confined to the vulva and/or perineum with a diameter >2 cm and no lymph node metastases
Stage III Lesions of any size extending to the lower urethra, vagina or anus and/or unilateral node metastases
Stage IVa Lesions invading upper urethra, bladder, rectum or pelvic bone with or without bilateral positive groin nodes regardless of extent of primary
Stage IVb Any distant metastases including pelvic lymph nodes.

TREATMENT OF INVASIVE SQUAMOUS CELL CARCINOMA

Surgical treatment

The standard treatment is radical vulvectomy and bilateral lymphadenectomy (but not routinely of the pelvic nodes).

- Three separate incisions are used to remove the tumour and the groin lymph nodes. Wide local excision of smaller tumours with separate node dissections can be used. With small laterally-placed tumours ipsilateral node dissection alone may be possible.

- Primary closure of the wound can usually be obtained by undermining the skin flaps but tension on the suture lines at the closure junction is almost inevitable. Rotational skin flaps improve healing and cosmetic results.
- The major postoperative complications are wound infection, wound breakdown and lymphocyst collection in the groins. Late complications involve tumour recurrence (about 10%), chronic lymphoedema and profound psychosexual disturbance.

The 5-year survival rate of women treated surgically is 75% with no node involvement, and 40% with node involvement.

Radiotherapy
Radiotherapy is most commonly used as an adjuvant (planned extra) treatment for the groins in patients with positive groin lymph nodes.
- Vulval cancer is susceptible to radiotherapy but normal vulval skin is exquisitely sensitive resulting in severe side-effects such as moist desquamation, ulceration and fibrosis. This can often prevent full treatment.
- Pre-operative irradiation may reduce the size of primary lesions and make operation possible.

Treatment of advanced lesions is difficult and accompanied by a poor prognosis.

Basal cell carcinoma
- Usually occurs on the labia majora, beginning as a small nodule which becomes ulcerated centrally (rodent ulcer).
- Lymphatics are not involved and local excision is usually adequate.
- The coexistence of an invasive squamous carcinoma within the lesions must be excluded.

Melanoma
- Arise from pigmented naevi. Prophylactic excision of pigmented vulvar naevi is recommended because they are usually symptomless even after they have become malignant.
- Treatment is by wide local excision and removal of any affected nodes because more radical procedures did not improve recurrence rates or survival.

Sarcoma
- This is a rare lesion. The mean age of patients with sarcoma is about 40 years.
- Treatment is by extensive local excision but the benefit of lymphadenectomy is unclear. Distant recurrence is common.

Bartholin's gland tumours

- These are rare lesions which may be adenocarcinoma (45%), squamous carcinoma (40%), sarcoma (5%), melanoma (1%) or undifferentiated (the remainder).
- Diagnosis is usually late because of the deep site of origin and the tumours may present with ulceration of the vulva and vagina.
- Treatment is by extensive local excision accompanied by inguinal and pelvic lymphadenectomy.
- The 5-year survival rate is probably under 10%.

FURTHER READING

Burghardt E (ed) 1993 Surgical gynecological oncology. Thieme Medical Publications, Stuttgart

Coppleson M 1992 Gynecologic oncology, 2nd edn, Vol 1. Churchill Livingstone, Edinbugh

McKay M 1995 Vulval dermatoses. Clinical obstetrics and gynaecology 34:614–629. Lippincott, Philadelphia

MacLean A B 1995 Lichen sclerosus. Personal Assessment in Continuing Education (PACE). RCOG, London

Ridley C M, Oriel J D, Robinson A J 1992 Colour atlas of diseases of the vulva. Champman & Hall, London

Shepherd J J, Monaghan J M 1990 Clinical gynaecological oncology, 2nd edn. Blackwell Scientific, Oxford

Sonnex C, Sterling J 1996 Interface: managing vulval disease. British Journal of Sexual Medicine 23:14–18

VAGINAL DISCHARGE

PHYSIOLOGICAL

- The vaginal fluid is a transudate through the epithelium along with desquamated cells, some polymorphs, and bacterial flora, predominantly large Gram-positive bacilli (lactobacilli).
- Contributions to the fluid also come from the cervical mucus and secretions of Skene's and Bartholin's glands. The vaginal fluid is highly acidic due to the lactic acid from the lactobacilli and glycogen from the desquamated cells.
- The acid pH of the vagina and its normal bacterial flora are among the factors which provide natural defence mechanisms for the lower genital tract.
- Among the factors which impair the defence mechanisms are:
  - —age—infection more liable to occur during childhood and after the menopause
  - —menstrual cycle—the alkalinity of the secretions around menses makes infection more likely
  - —pregnancy and the puerperium—a rise in pH encourages infection. Trauma at delivery with reduction in acidity by lochia and contamination with potentially pathogenic bowel flora makes the puerperium a time of particular susceptibility

—oestrogen-containing oral contraceptives increase the pH of vaginal fluid

—foreign bodies—objects such as beads or cotton wool in children or forgotten tampons in adults act as a focus for infection

—an IUD may produce a vaginal discharge due to chronic irritation of the endometrium.

The significance of a cervical ectropion

- The term 'cervical erosion' is a misnomer and should be abandoned.
- An ectropion is an area of columnar epithelium which has (or seems to have) extended beyond its normal boundaries.
- A cervical ectropion may therefore arise:
  —congenitally—the squamo-columnar junction lies on what should be the ectocervix
  —secondary to oestrogen-containing oral contraceptives
  —as a result of delivery—the squamo-columnar junction is normally sited but the parous cervix is patulous. (*Note*: the bivalve speculum may open the closed parous cervix and falsely give an impression of ectropion.)
- Vaginal discharge may be augmented by an increased secretion of mucus from a cervical ectropion.
- It is not to be confused with chronic cervicitis (see p. 263).

PATHOLOGICAL

Infections with *C. albicans* and *T. vaginalis* form up to 90% of pruritic vaginal discharges.

Candida infections

Clinical features

- Intense pruritus and soreness which may worsen in the evening and at night
- Thick, white discharge (like curdled milk) adherent to the vaginal skin
- Erythema of the vagina and labia minora which may extend perianally and onto the thighs
- The fungus is often carried in the gastrointestinal tract and/or the mouth
- The vagina is frequently infected via the perineum but minor trauma (e.g. intercourse) facilitates infection.

Predisposing factors

- Pregnancy—candidal vaginitis is the commonest of all infections in pregnancy. Between 15 and 20% of pregnant women may be affected
- Menstrual cycle—growth of *Candida* is promoted at the end of the luteal phase

- Medical disorders such as diabetes mellitus (marked increase) and iron deficiency anaemia
- Drugs: oestrogen-containing oral contraceptives; broad-spectrum antibiotics; corticosteroids; immunosuppressive agents
- Clothing—e.g. occlusive tights.

Diagnosis
- Clinical features—examine the vagina directly
- Microscopy of the discharge suspended in a drop of normal saline—mycelial filaments and spores will be visible
- Culture on glucose agar of swabs obtained in Stuart's transport medium.

Treatment
- Fungicidal drugs, e.g. nystatin or one of the imidazoles vaginally or fluconazole orally; effectiveness is >80%
- Genital hygiene—daily washing with bland soap and water is all that is necessary
- Clothing—avoidance of close-fitting tights; washing of underwear at >80°C.

Trichomonal infections
- Caused by *Trichomonas vaginalis*—a flagellated protozoon.
- They are usually sexually transmitted, and they may mask the presence (and the spread) of gonococcal infections.
- Cervical cytology can be highly abnormal in the presence of *T. vaginalis* (see p. 266). The cervical smear must be repeated after adequate treatment of the infection.

Clinical features
- Itching and/or burning sensation with dyspareunia
- Frothy vaginal discharge (pH 5–6) which may be white, green or brownish. The 'typical' appearance is due to gaseous fermentation by a commensal aerogenic streptococcus
- Some vulval oedema and congestion. Erythema is less marked than in *Candida* infections
- The vaginal skin is reddish-purple, perhaps with dark-red spots seen best at colposcopy.

Diagnosis
- Clinical features—examine the vagina directly; the vaginal pH is alkaline (pH 5–6)
- Microscopy of the discharge suspended in a drop of normal saline—motile flagellated protozoa are seen (about the same size as a polymorph leukocyte)
- Culture of swabs collected in Bushby's brown transport medium.

Treatment
Metronidazole for both partners.

Gonococcal infections

These are due to *Neisseria gonorrhoeae*. This bacterium attacks columnar and transitional epithelium, e.g. in the urethra, para-urethral ducts and glands, endocervix and anorectal canal.

Clinical features

- Painful swelling of the vulva
- Dysuria and frequency due to urethritis
- Greenish vaginal discharge 2–7 days (or longer) after intercourse with infected partner
- Vaginal skin red and oedematous
- Purulent exudate from the urethra and cervix
- Salpingo-oophoritis may develop (see p. 230).

Diagnosis

- Clinical features and history of contacts
- Gram staining of purulent exudates—*N. gonorrhoeae* are Gram-negative intra- and extracellular diplococci (i.e. they appear in pairs)
- Swabs from potentially infected sites. The full range for accurate sampling is endocervix, urethra, rectum and throat
- High vaginal swabs are of no value in most cases
- Culture by direct inoculation on modified Thayer–Martin plates. Swabs can be transported to the laboratory in Stuart's transport medium.

Treatment

- *Penicillin-sensitive organisms*: use oral probenecid; then procaine penicillin (i.m.) *or* oral ampicillin
- *β-lactamase-producing penicillin-resistant organisms*: use co-amoxiclav, erythromycin or, if necessary, spectinomycin
- *Patients allergic to penicillin*: use erythromycin or spectinomycin
- Contacts must be followed up.

Bacterial vaginosis

This is due to *Gardnerella vaginalis*, various anaerobic species and the motile bacilli of the *Mobiluncus* species.

Clinical features

- The characteristic symptom is an offensive 'fishy' vaginal discharge due to amines produced by the organisms. This is very distressing to the patient.
- Inflammation or irritation are not common.
- *Gardnerella vaginalis* is also found in over 20% of healthy, symptomless women.
- Bacterial vaginosis, perhaps as a co-infection with *Ureaplasma urealyticum* and *Mycoplasma hominis*, has been implicated in causing chorio-amnionitis and pre-term labour.

Diagnosis
- A drop of 10% potassium hydroxide added to a sample of the discharge on a glass slide releases the fishy odour.
- Microscopy of a wet film shows the motile *Mobiluncus* species.

Treatment
Metronidazole.

Infections with other organisms
- All pyogenic organisms can become pathogenic after trauma, in the presence of a foreign body, or after delivery.
- *Pediculosis pubis* is usually transmitted sexually and scabies can be: therefore check for other STDs if either is found.
- Vulvo-vaginitis may arise due to infestation with amoebae, schistosomes, or threadworms.

BENIGN CONDITIONS OF THE VAGINA AND CERVIX

GAERTNER DUCT CYSTS

- These arise from the mesonephric (Wolffian) duct and therefore occur antero-laterally in the vagina.
- They may be single or multiple and of varied size.
- Histology shows a single layer of cuboidal epithelium.
- Treatment is by excision or marsupialisation.

VAGINAL INCLUSION CYSTS

Usually small and often multiple, resulting from inversion of small fragments of vaginal skin after delivery or vaginal surgery.

ENDOMETRIOSIS (see p. 197)

CONDYLOMATA ACUMINATA

- Genital warts are caused by papova (DNA) virus.
- They are sexually transmitted and therefore may be accompanied by other STDs.
- They grow larger in pregnancy and tend to regress after delivery.
- Treatment is by podophyllin (avoid in pregnancy), saturated trichloracetic acid or electrocautery. Severe cases can be destroyed by laser (under GA).

PAPILLOMAS OF VAGINA AND CERVIX

- Cervical papillomas are more common.
- Clinically they can be difficult to differentiate from genital warts.
- They derive from the squamous epithelium with various degrees of keratinisation. The stalk is of fibrous connective tissue.
- They need to be removed surgically and sent for histological examination because of their malignant potential.

OTHER (RARE) BENIGN TUMOURS—e.g. fibroleiomyoma

CHRONIC CERVICITIS

- This is characterised by a hypertrophied, spongy cervix, in parous women presenting with seemingly purulent vaginal discharge.
- An ectropion (p. 259) may be present and/or several small or large retention cysts of the cervical mucous glands (Nabothian follicles).
- If treatment is necessary it can be carried out in outpatients using cryocautery.

CERVICAL POLYP

The commonest lesion of the cervix.
- It is a smooth, pedunculated growth from the columnar epithelium of the endocervix.
- Polyps can be due to hypertrophy of the mucous membrane or may be true benign neoplasms.
- The surface epithelium of the polyp is often ulcerated, causing the intermenstrual bleeding with which patients most commonly present.
- Cervical polyps are of low malignant potential but rarely a seemingly innocent polyp is the early lesion of sarcoma botryoides.
- They can be avulsed by twisting and, if necessary, the base can be cauterised.
- Histological examination should also be carried out.

INTRAEPITHELIAL NEOPLASIA OF THE VAGINA AND CERVIX

Nomenclature and definitions

Dyskaryosis—a cytological term which refers to abnormalities of individual cells such as enlargement and hyperchromasia of the nuclei with uneven chromatin distribution, irregular nuclear membrane and multinucleation. It is graded mild, moderate or severe: see Table 23.1.

Dysplasia—a histological diagnosis which describes abnormalities of epithelium. It is defined as a lesion in which part of the thickness of the epithelium is replaced by cells showing varying degrees of atypia.

Carcinoma-in-situ refers to lesions in which all or most of the epithelium shows the following features:
   —loss of stratification and polarity throughout the full thickness of the epithelium
   —variation in size and shape of cells
   —increased nuclear/cytoplasmic ratio

—frequent bizarre mitoses
—the basement membrane is intact.

The only difference between dysplasia and carcinoma-in-situ is one of degree. Both these terms have now been replaced by the term **intraepithelial neoplasia**.

Table 23.1   Cervical epithelial neoplasia

Cytology	Grade	Histology
Mild dyskaryosis	1	Mild dysplasia
Moderate dyskaryosis	2	Moderate dysplasia
Severe dyskaryosis	3	Severe dysplasia and carcinoma-in-situ

VAGINAL INTRAEPITHELIAL NEOPLASIA (VAIN)

VAIN is asymptomatic and detected only by cytological and/or colposcopic examination.
- Its appearances are as for CIN (see below).
- The treatment options for VAIN are:
  —laser vaporisation
  —surgical excision
  —radiation (rarely)
  —intravaginal 5-fluorouracil (rarely).
- *NO patient with an abnormal smear should have a hysterectomy without prior colposcopy because CIN extends onto the vaginal walls in approximately 4% of women. If a hysterectomy is being performed in the presence of CIN all the affected epithelium must be excised with the hysterectomy specimen.*
- When VAIN is detected following hysterectomy, management is difficult because the angles of the vagina are difficult to assess by cytology and colposcopy.
- Discrete areas of VAIN away from the vaginal vault can be laser vaporised; areas involving the vaginal vault hysterectomy scar are treated by upper vaginectomy.

CERVICAL INTRAEPITHELIAL NEOPLASIA—CIN

Aetiology
- CIN and cervical cancer have the same origin.
- Approximately 30–50% of cases of CIN will, if left untreated, progress to invasive disease.

Epidemiology
- CIN and cervical cancer are sexually transmitted diseases.

Associated characteristics of affected women include number of sexual partners, divorce, venereal disease and religious or cultural factors.

- Although the common denominator appears to be age at first intercourse, the majority of affected women are not promiscuous and should not be stigmatised.
- A male factor is also involved. The wives of men with prostatic or penile cancer have a higher risk of cervical cancer.
- Cervical neoplasia is most common among lower socioeconomic groups.
- Prolonged use of oral contraception and cigarette smoking are associated with an increased risk of cervical neoplasia.
- The age-specific prevalence for CIN 1 and CIN 2 is 20–29 years, and for CIN 3 it is 36–39 years.

Biology
- The *transformation zone (TZ)* is a circumferential region of tissue between the vaginal (squamous) and endocervical (columnar) tissue. It is composed of columnar epithelium which has descended onto the ectocervix, although the border between the columnar and squamous epithelium is usually not finally defined until adult life.
- The columnar epithelium of the TZ undergoes metaplasia to squamous epithelium to a varying degree. This active process exposes the epithelium to neoplastic transformation.
- The precise mutagen involved is not proven but human papillomavirus (HPV) types 16, 18, 31 and 33 are found in over 90% of invasive cervical cancers.

CYTOLOGICAL SCREENING AND THE PREVENTION OF CERVICAL CANCER

- The success of cytological screening programmes depends on the percentage of women at risk screened.
- Comprehensive programmes have achieved significant reductions in both the incidence of, and death rate from, the disease. The remaining unscreened women at risk have a much greater risk of having (and dying from) the disease.
- The number of women screened and the frequency of screening depends on the resources available. One recommended screening policy is as follows:
  —the first smear should be taken at 20 years of age
  —thereafter intervals of 3–5 years are adequate
  —regular testing can stop from 64 years of age if previous smears have been normal.
- Currently over 80% of women in Britain are screened.
- The incidence of cervical cancer is beginning to fall and cancer deaths are expected to follow suit.

CERVICAL SMEARS

- The correlation between the level of dyskaryosis in a smear and the grade of CIN is not exact (approximately 70% agreement).
- Cervical smears are graded by assessment of individual cell morphology and recommendations are made as follows:
  - **inadequate**—insufficient cellular material for assessment; repeat smear required
  - **negative**—no abnormal cells seen; repeat in recommended screening interval (usually 3 or 5 years)
  - **borderline**—minor cellular changes; repeat and refer for colposcopy if persists on two or three occasions
  - **mild dyskaryosis**—superficial cell (mild); nuclear abnormalities with abundant cytoplasm and angular cell borders. Repeat smear and refer for colposcopy if persists
  - **moderate dyskaryosis**—intermediate cell (moderate); nucleus much larger in proportion to the whole cell than normally but occupying less than 50% of the cell. Refer for colposcopy
  - **severe dyskaryosis**—parabasal cell (severe); the nucleus occupies more than 50% of the cell. The cell border is round or oval. Refer *urgently* for colposcopy
  - **severe dyskaryosis? invasive**—severe dyskaryosis plus cells suggestive of invasion. Refer *urgently* for colposcopy
  - **glandular neoplasia**—atypical columnar type cells suggestive of dysplasia of the endocervical columnar epithelium: cervical glandular intraepithelial neoplasia (CGIN). Refer for colposcopy.

Histological characteristics of CIN grades

CIN 1 (mild dysplasia)
- Upper two thirds of epithelium exhibits relatively good differentiation
- Minor nuclear abnormalities
- Few mitotic figures confined to basal third.

CIN 2 (moderate dysplasia)
- Upper half of epithelium is well differentiated
- Moderate nuclear abnormalities
- Mitotic figures (some abnormal) present in basal two thirds

CIN 3 (severe dysplasia/carcinoma in situ)
- Maturation confined to superficial one third of epithelium or absent
- Nuclear abnormalities marked and throughout full thickness
- Mitotic figures may be numerous, at all levels and with many abnormal configurations.

Taking and processing of cervical smears

- The proper taking, interpretation and follow-up of cervical smears are fundamental to the whole screening programme.
- The cervix must be inspected carefully. The presence of a suspicious abnormality requires referral urgently for colposcopy irrespective of the smear result.
- Specimens for cervical and/or vaginal cytology are usually taken with a wooden (or plastic) Ayre spatula.
- All smears must be accompanied by adequate information about the patient.
- *False-negative smears* are those reported as normal in a patient who has a neoplastic lesion of the cervix. This may be due to:
  —an error in taking the smear—cervix not properly sampled
  —technical problem—smear too thin, too thick, too bloody, poorly fixed or poorly stained
  —diagnostic failures—misinterpretation by the cytologist
  —the size of the lesion (too small) so that very few cells exfoliate.
- The reported frequency of false-negative smears is between 1.8 and 20%!
- *False-positive smears* are those in which malignant changes are seen but subsequent full examination of the cervix fails to reveal them.
- They may be due to errors in the laboratory; therefore positive smears should be repeated before any surgery is contemplated.
- However, the cytologist may be correct and the source of the malignant cells may have remained undetected higher in the cervical canal and finally been detected at colposcopy or even cone biopsy.

EVALUATION OF THE PATIENT WITH ABNORMAL CERVICAL CYTOLOGY

- In the majority of patients with CIN the cervix will look quite normal to the naked eye.
- No patient with cytological evidence of CIN should be treated without prior colposcopic assessment. Colposcopy is the detailed examination of the cervix using binocular magnification and bright illumination. The aims of colposcopic examination of the cervix in women with CIN are:
  —to demarcate the boundaries of the transformation zone (TZ)
  —to rule out invasive disease by directed biopsies
  —to confirm/refute the suspicion raised by cytology
  —to plan appropriate treatment.

TREATMENT OF CIN

Intraepithelial neoplasia is a localised problem and can be treated satisfactorily by excision or destruction of the abnormal epithelium. The method used is less important than the assurance that all neoplastic tissue is destroyed or removed. The suggested methods of treatment include loop diathermy excision of TZ, cone biopsy, local destruction of the whole TZ, and hysterectomy.

Loop diathermy excision of TZ
- This can often be carried out as an outpatient.
- A major benefit over destructive methods discussed below is that the area removed is available for histology.
- Because of its ease of use, safety and cheapness it is now the commonest form of treatment.

Cone biopsy
- Traditionally performed with a knife under general anaesthesia, this can be done under local anaesthesia using a modified loop diathermy technique.
- It can provide both firm diagnosis and comprehensive treatment. It is even more effective if colposcopically directed (99% primary cure rate).
- The operation is not without immediate or longer-term hazard such as:
  —primary or secondary haemorrhage
  —local infection
  —cervical stenosis (small cones)
  —cervical incompetence (large cones).
- Fertility is probably unaffected, but mid-trimester abortion and pre-term delivery may be more common and possibly directly related to the size of the cone removed.
- If the raw area of the cervix is covered by mobilising the remainder of the cervical epithelium, residual CIN in the endocervical crypts may be covered and remain occult.
- Apparent incomplete excision may require further definitive surgery (e.g. another cone biopsy, or hysterectomy) in approximately one third of cases.

Local destruction of the whole TZ
- This can be achieved by carbon dioxide laser, cold coagulation, cryocautery, radical electrocoagulation diathermy, or electrocautery.
- These have the advantage that they are not associated with significant morbidity (including fertility-related problems). In addition, laser, cryocautery and cold coagulation may be performed as outpatient procedures with or without local anaesthesia.
- Before selecting a patient for a local destructive technique or diathermy excision the patient must be assessed by a competent colposcopist who:
  —is able to see the lesion and the transformation zone in its entirety

—is certain that there is no evidence of invasion by taking colposcopically directed biopsies

—is certain that there is no suspicion (cytologically or colposcopically) of abnormal columnar cells suggesting an endometrial neoplasm

—is assured that there will be regular cytological and colposcopic follow-up.

Hysterectomy
- This may be the method of choice for CIN 3 in women who have completed their family, who wish complete assurance of cure, and/or in whom follow-up is likely to be difficult.
- Removal of a cuff of vagina is not necessary.

CARCINOMA OF THE VAGINA

Primary malignant tumours of the vagina are rare, and an invasive lesion is more likely to be due to secondary spread.

SQUAMOUS CELL CARCINOMA

- This is the commonest histological type and accounts for 1–2% of all gynaecological malignancies.
- Most occur between the ages of 55 and 70 years with a peak incidence of about 65 years.
- The commonest presenting symptoms are vaginal discharge, and bleeding as a result of ulceration of the tumour. The most frequent site is the posterior vaginal wall.

Staging
Stage 0: Intraepithelial carcinoma
Stage I: Limited to vaginal wall
Stage II: Outside the vagina but not to pelvic side walls
Stage III: To the pelvic side walls and/or symphysis pubis
Stage IV: Extension beyond the true pelvis or involving the bladder or rectum.
  The lesions are usually moderately undifferentiated.
  Tumours in the lower third of the vagina spread to the inguinal nodes like carcinoma of the vulva (p. 254). In the upper vagina, spread is similar to that of carcinoma of the cervix (p. 270).

Treatment
Radiotherapy is the treatment of choice unless the lesion is at the introitus, when radical surgery may be possible. Five-year survival rates are: Stage I 85%; Stage II 55%; Stage III 30%; Stage IV <10%.

ADENOCARCINOMA

- This rare tumour is most often found in association with vaginal

adenosis in young women with a history of intrauterine exposure to diethyl stilboestrol (DES).
- The most frequent histological type is a clear cell adenocarcinoma, and the commonest site is the upper third of the vagina.
- Spread is by local extension and by the lymphatics and bloodstream.

Staging
As for squamous carcinoma of the cervix.

Treatment
- Radical hysterectomy, vaginectomy and pelvic lymphadenectomy are preferred.
- Radiotherapy can be used if expert surgery is not available, or in young women with small lesions (because the remainder of the vagina, adjacent structures and ovarian function can be preserved).
- Five-year survival rates are: Stage I 80%; Stage II <20%; Stages III and IV none.

SECONDARY VAGINAL TUMOURS
- Metastatic carcinoma of the vagina is commoner than a primary cancer.
- It occurs frequently in carcinoma of the cervix, sometimes after carcinoma of the endometrium and occasionally in carcinoma of the ovary or choriocarcinoma. It may rarely follow hypernephroma or carcinoma of the colon or rectum.

CARCINOMA OF THE CERVIX
- Cervical cancer is second to ovarian as the commonest malignant tumour of the genital tract, comprising 30% of the total.
- Despite an overall fall in incidence, particularly among older women, the peak age is still 50–59 years.
- However, in the past two decades the incidence has doubled in women under 40 years and the mortality has almost trebled in women under 34 years of age.
- This worrying rise may have halted in well-screened populations.
- The epidemiology is as for CIN.
- 75% of the tumours are squamous, approximately 15% are adenosquamous and 10% are adenocarcinoma.
  Adenocarcinomas are becoming relatively more common.

SQUAMOUS CARCINOMA
Histology
- Cell characteristics:
  —loss of stratification

—various degrees of immaturity and lack of differentiation
—pleomorphism of cells and nuclei
—hyperchromatic nuclei
—abundant and atypical mitoses
—giant cell formation.
- Architecture:
  —the malignant epithelium has broken through the basement membrane
  —lymphocyte and polymorph infiltration of stroma. The more immature and undifferentiated the tumour, the more malignant it is (and more radiosensitive).

Spread
- Early spread occurs by local infiltration.
- Upward spread into the body of the uterus is uncommon, and forward spread into the bladder occurs late. Obstruction of the ureters is common (many deaths occur due to uraemia).
- Lymphatic spread first involves a primary group of nodes:
  —Parametrial   —Hypogastric
  —Vesico-vaginal   —Obturator
  —Recto-vaginal   —External iliac

and then a secondary group of nodes:
  —Sacral   —Vaginal (deep and superficial)
  —Common iliac   —Para-aortic
- Even in clinically assessed stage Ib disease pelvic lymph nodes will be affected in about 15% of patients.

Clinical features
- Cervical cancer may be asymptomatic (even to a late stage) and be detected by routine cervical smear or examination.
- Intermenstrual, postmenopausal or postcoital bleeding are the commonest presenting symptoms. Vaginal discharge is less frequent and a later development.
- Pain occurs only in the very late stages.
- On examination the cervix may:
  —appear normal (e.g. intraepithelial or endocervical)
  —be hard with a granular 'erosion' which bleeds to touch
  —be ulcerated.
- Moderately advanced growths may be exophytic (polypoid), infiltrative or ulcerative.

Management
- *Close cooperation between gynaecologist and radiotherapist is vital.*
- Check full blood count, urea, and electrolytes.
- Carry out chest X-ray and excretion urography (IVP). A bone survey for metastasis is not routine. The value of lymphangiography remains controversial.

Conditions of the lower genital tract

- Carry out pelvic examination (vaginal and rectal) under anaesthesia to assess the extent of the disease. This is the definitive staging (see information box) which allows comparison of treatment results.
- Proceed to:
  —cervical biopsy for histology
  —cystoscopy—looking for bullous oedema which suggests involvement of the underlying muscle. (The first insertion of caesium can be carried out at this time if need be.)

Carcinoma of cervix: clinical staging

Stage 0:	Intraepithelial carcinoma (p. 264)
Stage I:	Invasive carcinoma confined to the cervix
Stage Ia1:	No lesion visible at clinical examination, and stromal invasion is less than 3 mm (microinvasion)
Stage Ia2:	Stromal invasion between 3 and 5 mm with maximum lateral spread of 7 mm
Stage Ib:	All other stage I lesions
Stage Ib1:	Clinical lesions no greater than 4 cm in size
Stage Ib2:	Clinical lesions >4 cm in size
Stage II:	The carcinoma extends beyond the cervix but not to the pelvic side wall; and/or the upper two thirds of the vagina are involved
Stage IIa:	No parametrial involvement
Stage IIb:	Obvious parametrial involvement
Stage III:	The carcinoma extends to the pelvic side wall and/or the lower one third of the vagina is involved. Presence of hydronephrosis or non-functioning kidney
Stage IIIa:	No extension to the pelvic wall but involvement of the lower third of vagina
Stage IIIb:	Extension to the pelvic wall or hydronephrosis or non-functioning kidney
Stage IV:	The carcinoma extends beyond the true pelvis or involves the bladder or rectum (bullous oedema is excluded)
Stage IVa:	Spread of tumour onto adjacent pelvic organs
Stage IVb:	Spread to distant organs

TREATMENT OF STAGE IA1 (MICRO-INVASIVE) CARCINOMA

Working definition

A micro-invasive lesion is one in which the carcinoma invades the stroma in one or more places to a depth of 3 mm or less below the basement membrane and in which lymphatics and blood vessels cannot be seen to be involved.

The following qualifications are necessary:

- it is not possible to examine the whole specimen histologically in every case

- it is difficult to distinguish extensive gland or cleft involvement from stromal invasion
- if clumps of tumour cells can be seen in vascular spaces, even if invasion is minimal, lymph nodes are involved in up to 25% of cases.

Treatment
- Conservative therapy by cone biopsy can be considered in young women who are anxious to retain fertility. *Close cytological and colposcopic follow-up is vital.*
- Simple hysterectomy should be used:
  —for older women or in those whose family is complete
  —when the pathologist is uncertain of the diagnosis of micro-invasion.

  A cuff of vagina should be taken if the transformation zone extends onto the vagina.

- Radical therapy (as for stage Ib) may be best for those with clumps of tumour cells in vascular spaces, and certainly if stromal invasion is more than 3 mm (stage Ia2).

The cure rate should be close to 100%.

TREATMENT OF STAGES IB AND IIA

The choice is between radical (Wertheim's) hysterectomy and radiotherapy.

Radical hysterectomy
- The lesion most suitable for treatment by radical hysterectomy is one which is confined to the cervix or with only minimal extension beyond it, particularly in the younger patient.
- The procedure involves removal of the uterus, cervix, parametria, upper one third to one half of the vagina and as many pelvic lymph nodes as possible.
- It is now thought unnecessary to sacrifice ovaries routinely; this is a great advantage, particularly in younger women.

Advantages of surgery
- The tumour is removed, which patients find psychologically reassuring.
- Treatment is less prolonged.
- The ovaries need not be removed in young patients with early disease.
- Early and late complications of radiotherapy are avoided.
- Infection is no bar to treatment (unlike radiotherapy).
- Potential radio-resistance is overcome.
- More prognostic information is available.
- Follow-up examination and radiological monitoring is easier.
- Local recurrence is treatable with radiotherapy.

Disadvantages of surgery
- Only selected patients benefit from it.
- Bladder dysfunction is common.
- The vagina is shortened.

Complications of surgery
Immediate and short-term: e.g. anaesthetic problems, haemorrhage, shock, sepsis, thromboembolism
Long-term: e.g. urinary retention, ureteric and rectal fistulae, lymphocyst—a collection of lymph on the pelvic side wall.

Radiotherapy
- The tumour itself and any paracervical spread are attacked using intrauterine and intravaginal caesium 137.
- The pelvic lymph nodes and their lymphatics are dealt with mainly by external irradiation.
- The aim is to deliver 60–75 Gy at point A (2 cm lateral to the midline; 2 cm above the lateral fornix in the same sagittal plane as the uterus). Point B (5 cm from the midline at the same level and the same place) receives only 25% of the dosage according to the inverse square law. External irradiation (preferably by linear accelerator) should deliver 50–70 Gy to the pelvic side walls.
- There is considerable variation in individual policies and regimes but the overall aims are the same.

Complications of radiotherapy
- Vaginal stenosis may develop in up to 85% of irradiation patients. This can be minimised by regular sexual intercourse or the use of vaginal dilators. Dyspareunia is common.
- Radiation-induced menopause is inevitable. This can be managed by topical or systemic oestrogen replacement.
- Urinary tract injuries may occur. Some frequency and dysuria is inevitable. Bladder ulcers can be difficult to cure. Vesico-vaginal fistulae occur rarely and usually some 3–8 months after treatment.
- Uretero-vaginal fistulae are more liable to occur when radiotherapy and surgery are combined. Surgical correction of fistulae is difficult; urinary diversion is usually required.
- Intestinal complications may arise, varying from diarrhoea to rectal fistulae.
- Local recurrence is difficult to treat. Chemotherapy is ineffective but selected patients can be saved by extensive surgery (pelvic exenteration).
- Follow-up is difficult due to the fibrosis induced in the pelvis by radiotherapy.
- Occasionally radiotherapy causes secondary cancers many years later.

Combined radiotherapy and surgery

- Radiotherapy was formerly given pre-operatively but this is rarely done now because there is no demonstrable benefit and it alters the histological appearances of the specimen.
- Adjuvant (planned additional) radiotherapy is given postoperatively if more than two lymph nodes are involved or if the excision margins of the tumour are incomplete.

Note: if invasive carcinoma is diagnosed as a result of cone biopsy, definitive treatment should, if possible, be deferred for 6 weeks to allow healing to occur. Otherwise the complications of radiotherapy and/or surgery are increased.

Chemotherapy

Combination chemotherapy (e.g. cisplatin, methotrexate, bleomycin) is given to fit patients with proven systemic disease. Tumour partial response is common and survival is lengthened. Cure is uncommon. Chemotherapy is used as palliation (e.g. to relieve pain due to tumour pressing on nerve roots).

Results of treatment

- Whatever the method used to treat carcinoma of the cervix, the 5-year survival rates are comparable at:
  —Stage Ib 85–90%
  —Stage IIa 70–75% (if lymph nodes are positive, survival drops to 50–60%).
- The results of surgery improve and its complications lessen with the expertise of the surgeon. This condition is probably best fulfilled by sub-specialists in regional cancer centres.
- To ensure the best treatment for each patient the following *minimum* criteria must be met:
  —there must be close cooperation between the surgical and radiotherapeutic teams
  —any surgery should be carried out by, or under the guidance of, a gynaecologist adequately trained in radical surgery and able to cope with any contingency
  —close follow-up must be organised.

TREATMENT OF CARCINOMA OF THE CERVIX—STAGES IIB TO IV

- The treatment of choice is radiotherapy.
- Pelvic exenteration is applicable when radiotherapy is unlikely to be effective or when the tumour has not regressed during radiotherapy.
  —*Anterior exenteration*—bladder removed in conjunction with radical hysterectomy and lymphadenectomy
  —*Posterior exenteration*—rectum removed
  —*Total exenteration*—both bladder and rectum removed.

- *These operations are justified only if there is some expectation of useful life as a result.* They are not applicable if extra-pelvic metastases are present.
- A terminal colostomy and ileal conduit are to be preferred to a 'wet' colostomy.
- Five-year survival rates are as follows: Stage IIb 50–60%; Stage III 30–35%; Stage IV <10%.

RECURRENT CARCINOMA OF THE CERVIX

- If the tumour recurs it usually does so within 18 months of treatment. The main sites are:
  —deep pelvis: 35%
  —distant spread: 30%
  —lateral pelvis: 15%
  —bladder or rectum: 10%
  —central pelvis: 10%.
- The most frequent signs and symptoms are:
  —renewed vaginal bleeding
  —pain
  —weight loss
  —evidence of urinary tract obstruction.
- If radiotherapy has not been used, or was incomplete, then further treatment is possible.
- Occasionally exenteration can be carried out.
- Palliation is usually all that can be offered.
- For relief of pain in advanced cancer see page 293.
- The ultimate causes of death, in order of frequency, are uraemia, cachexia, severe haemorrhage, complications of treatment and, rarely, remote metastases to vital organs.

ADENOCARCINOMA OF THE CERVIX

- These tumours are rare but they tend to grow and spread as squamous carcinoma.
- Treatment is as for squamous carcinoma. They respond equally to radiotherapy or surgery.

FURTHER READING

Anderson M C, Jordan J, Morse A, Sharp F 1992 A text and atlas of integrated colposcopy. Chapman & Hall, London

Burghardt E (ed) 1993 Surgical gynecological oncology. Thieme Medical Publications, Stuttgart

Cartier R 1985 Practical colposcopy, 2nd edn. Laboratoire Cartier, Paris

Coppleson M 1992 Gynecologic oncology, 2nd edn, Vol 1. Churchill Livingstone, Edinburgh

Mould T, Singer A 1996 Prevention: cervical screening recent advances. British Journal of Sexual Medicine 23(1):6–10

Shepherd J J, Monaghan J M 1990 Clinical gynaecological oncology, 2nd edn. Blackwell Scientific, Oxford

24. Conditions of the body of the uterus and fallopian tubes

ENDOMETRIAL POLYPS (ADENOMA)

- These polyps are usually multiple before the menopause and may be a component of endometrial hyperplasia. After the menopause they are usually single (or few in number). They tend to recur.
- Most are symptomless but they may be associated with:
  —menorrhagia
  —intermenstrual bleeding
  —postcoital bleeding
  —postmenopausal bleeding.
- They are easily removed by small ovum forceps and curettage. Hysteroscopy may be of value also because a polyp may elude curettage.
- All polyps should be sent for histology to exclude malignant change.

UTERINE FIBROIDS

- A leiomyoma is a well-circumscribed benign uterine tumour derived mainly from smooth muscle but containing some fibrous connective tissue elements.
- It is the commonest tumour of the female genital tract, being present in at least 20% of women over the age of 35. The peak age incidence of symptoms is between 35 and 45 years.
- In Caucasian, but not Black, women they are associated with nulliparity or relative infertility.
- Growth may be related to oestrogen stimulation.

SITES OF ORIGIN

- Intramural – within uterine wall
- Subserous—projecting from the peritoneal surface of the uterus
- Intraligamentary—between the layers of the broad ligament
- Submucous—indenting the uterine cavity
- Cervical.

Submucous fibroids may become polypoidal and subserous ones pedunculated. Pedunculated fibroids may lose their uterine attachment and gain a secondary blood supply (parasitic fibroid).

GROSS CHARACTERISTICS

- Uterine fibroids may be small, medium-sized or large, and are usually multiple.
- They are usually firm, but can be soft and cystic if degeneration has taken place.
- They are white and characteristically whorled in appearance.
- There is a false capsule of compressed uterine muscle which allows easy enucleation (cf. adenomyosis).

HISTOLOGY

Groups and bundles of smooth muscle fibres are interlaced in twists and whorls. The fibrous component becomes more marked as the tumour enlarges.

CLINICAL FEATURES

- The majority are symptomless.
- Increased menstrual loss is usually caused by submucous fibroids. Intermenstrual bleeding may be due to a fibroid polyp with an ulcerated tip. (**Note**: Atypical menstrual symptoms may be due to a concurrent but separate pathology.)
- Pressure effects may give rise to bladder symptoms and interfere with venous return.
- Abdominal swelling may be noted.
- Pain is not a common symptom unless the fibroid has become complicated (see below).
- There is a rare association with polycythaemia.

DIFFERENTIAL DIAGNOSIS

- It must include all causes of pelvic swellings.
- It is not always easy to discern clinically between a solid ovarian tumour and a pedunculated fibroid.
- The difference between a fibroid and an adenomyoma may not be apparent until surgical removal is attempted.

Potential effects of fibroids on pregnancy
- Subfertility
- Abortion and pre-term labour
- Malpresentations
- Obstructed labour (rare)
- Third stage problems
- Delayed involution postpartum.

COMPLICATIONS OF FIBROIDS

- *Torsion of pedicle*
- *Haemorrhage*

- *Infection*—usually at the tip of a fibroid polyp
- *Hyaline degeneration*—present to some degree in most moderate to large-sized fibroids. The tumour may be painful, enlarged and soft. Cystic degeneration follows
- *Red degeneration* (necrobiosis)—occurs typically during pregnancy and is due to infarction of the centre of the tumour during mid-pregnancy. Characteristically the fibroid suddenly enlarges and is painful and tender. It can be mistaken for placental abruption or any acute abdominal emergency. It is treated conservatively during pregnancy
- *Calcification*—usually seen postmenopausally and/or in pedunculated fibroids
- *Malignant change* (leiomyosarcoma—see p. 282) occurs in under 0.5% of cases. The fibroid may grow suddenly and be painful and tender. It is difficult to differentiate clinically from other degenerative changes.

TREATMENT

Conservative management is appropriate:
    —when the tumours are small, the diagnosis is certain and there are no symptoms
    —during pregnancy
    —near the menopause when there are no symptoms and the tumour is not enlarging.

The short-term use (no more than 6 months) of LHRH analogues needs to be studied further. They reduce the size of fibroids, which may be of benefit in:
    —those with contraindications to surgery
    —as an adjunct to surgery if fibroids are large.

Surgery is indicated if:
    —the fibroids are causing symptoms or are growing rapidly. They are larger than a size corresponding to a 16-week pregnancy
    —the diagnosis is in doubt
    —they are likely to complicate a future pregnancy.
- *Hysterectomy* is the definitive treatment.
- *Myomectomy* is indicated for those women who are subfertile, want more children or refuse to undergo hysterectomy.
- It may be possible to resect small submucous fibroids endoscopically.
- Rupture of a myomectomy scar during subsequent pregnancy or labour is very rare, and vaginal delivery is often possible.
- (Any fibroids found at caesarean section should usually be left undisturbed because of the risk of haemorrhage.)

ENDOMETRIAL CARCINOMA

- This tumour constitutes 25–30% of all gynaecological malignancies.
- The incidence is low before 40 years of age (4%), rises sharply until 55 years and then falls slightly. A greater proportion of women with endometrial carcinoma are postmenopausal than is the case in carcinoma of the cervix. 25% of cases are premenopausal.
- Nulliparous women are 2–3 times more likely to develop endometrial carcinoma than are parous women, although half the women with the disease will have had one or more pregnancies.
- There is no relationship with social class.
- There is an association with gross obesity, polycystic ovary syndrome, and possibly diabetes mellitus.

Pathology

- Usually adenocarcinoma, but there may be benign squamous elements (adenoacanthoma) or malignant squamous elements (adenosquamous).
- It may be diffuse or circumscribed.

Histology

- In most cases the diagnosis is clear-cut due to the disordered architecture, atypical glands, and abnormal activity and characteristics of the cells.
- Benign cystic glandular hyperplasia is not liable to become malignant, but atypical hyperplasia is, and removal of the uterus is recommended.
- Spread is direct within the endometrium and, to a lesser degree, into the myometrium. Penetration to the serosa is uncommon.
- Lymphatic spread is along the ovarian vessels to the para-aortic nodes or through the myometrium and cervix to the pelvic nodes.

Clinical features

- Irregular vaginal bleeding—intermenstrual or postmenopausal
- Watery vaginal discharge may be present in postmenopausal women
- Abdominal and pelvic examination are unremarkable, except in late cases.

Population screening

- There is no certain method for screening the population at risk.
- Outpatient endometrial sampling is useful but not foolproof.
- Transvaginal ultrasound to measure endometrial thickness is non-invasive and quite accurate (thickness greater than 5 mm in postmenopausal women is abnormal).

INITIAL MANAGEMENT

- *Hysteroscopy and biopsy* should be carried out if endometrial carcinoma is suspected clinically or if the above tests are positive, suspicious or unsatisfactory.
- *Pre-operative evaluation* is as for carcinoma of the cervix (p. 270). Transvaginal ultrasound, MRI or CT scan may also be useful.
- *Pre-operative radiotherapy* does not improve the prognosis and makes histological grading of the tumour more difficult.
- *Total abdominal hysterectomy and bilateral salpingo-oophorectomy* is the operation of choice. Careful surgical staging is necessary, including:
  —aspiration of peritoneal fluid or peritoneal washings
  —palpation and inspection of all peritoneal structures
  —palpation with biopsy of pelvic and para-aortic lymph nodes.

Some surgeons take a cuff of vagina to reduce the chance of vaginal vault recurrence. The role of extensive node dissection (as for cancer of the cervix) is controversial.

Endometrial carcinoma: staging

Staging is surgical

Stage 0:	Atypical hyperplasia suspicious of malignancy
Stage I:	Carcinoma confined to the body of the uterus
Stage Ia:	Tumour limited to the endometrium
Stage Ib:	Invasion to < half myometrium
Stage Ic:	Invasion to > half myometrium but not reaching serosa
Stage II:	Carcinoma involving the body and cervix
Stage IIa:	Endocervical gland involvement only
Stage IIb:	Cervical stroma involvement
Stage III:	Carcinoma outside the uterus but not outside the true pelvis
Stage IIIa:	Tumour invades serosa and/or adnexa and/or positive peritoneal cytology
Stage IIIb:	Metastases to pelvic and/or para-aortic nodes
Stage IV:	Carcinoma involving the bladder or rectal mucosa (IVa) or outside the true pelvis (IVb)

Stage I is further subdivided according to the histology:

Grade 1:	Well differentiated tumour
Grade 2:	Differentiated tumour but with partly solid areas
Grade 3:	Undifferentiated tumour or predominantly solid

Further management

- Low-risk patients (i.e. stage Ia and Ib with G1 or G2 tumours) usually require no further therapy.
- Some surgeons perform radical hysterectomy (as carcinoma of the cervix) for stage II disease. Adjuvant radiotherapy may be

indicated in patients at high risk of recurrence but there is great variation in their selection.
- Results from cytotoxic therapy are disappointing.
- Recurrent disease can be treated with progestogens and/or radiotherapy. Pelvic exenteration is occasionally possible and a solitary vaginal vault lesion may be excisable.

Prognosis

The 5-year survival rate is:

Stage I: 80–85% (Grade 1 90%; Grade 3 65%)
Stage II: 55–60% (80% in best centres)
Stage III: 35–40% (60% in best centres)
Stage IV: <10% (15% in best centres).

SARCOMA OF THE UTERUS

These are rare tumours. Malignant degeneration in a leiomyoma accounts for half of them but they may arise from normal myometrium or endometrial stroma.

LEIOMYOSARCOMA

- Most patients are between 40 and 60 years of age.
- The commonest symptoms are abnormal vaginal bleeding and abdominal pain.
- A uterine mass is frequently palpable.
- Lymphatic spread is not common.
- Treatment is by total hysterectomy and bilateral salpingo-oophorectomy. Radiotherapy is relatively ineffective.

ENDOMETRIAL SARCOMA

- Most patients are between 50 and 70 years of age.
- Signs, symptoms and treatment are the same as for leiomyosarcoma.

SARCOMA BOTRYOIDES

- A rare tumour probably of mixed mesodermal origin usually occurring in children (any lesion in this age group should arouse suspicion).
- It is polypoidal, either single or multiple.
- Staging is as for carcinoma.
- Treatment combines chemotherapy with radiotherapy and then radical surgery (extended hysterectomy and vaginectomy).

Prognosis

The 5-year survival rate is about 45% for stage I disease and 30% in stage II.

CARCINOMA OF THE FALLOPIAN TUBE

- Primary tumours of the fallopian tube are exceedingly rare (0.3% of genital tract cancers).
- They tend to occur in women aged 40–60 years.
- The histology is papillary adenocarcinoma.
- The majority of patients will have had a watery vaginal discharge, and some will complain of abdominal pain. An abdominal mass may be palpable, but very few patients have all of these clinical features.
- Treatment is by total hysterectomy and bilateral salpingo-oophorectomy. External radiotherapy is applied afterwards, and chemotherapy can be used in some late cases.
- Five-year survival rates are between 5 and 25%, reflecting the lateness of diagnosis in most cases.

FURTHER READING

Burghardt E (ed) 1993 Surgical gynecological oncology. Thieme Medical Publications, Stuttgart

Coppleson M 1992 Gynecologic oncology, 2nd edn, Vol 2. Churchill Livingstone, Edinburgh

Shaw R W, Soutter W P, Stanton S L (eds) 1996 Gynaecology, 2nd edn. Churchill Livingstone, Edinburgh

Shepherd J J, Monaghan J M 1990 Clinical gynaecological oncology, 2nd edn. Blackwell Scientific, Oxford

Tindall V R 1990 Jeffcoate's principles of gynaecology, 5th edn. Butterworths, London

25. Conditions of the ovary

NON-NEOPLASTIC DISTENSION CYSTS

FOLLICULAR CYST(S) ('CYSTIC OVARY')

- Due to enlargement of one or more follicles which fail to rupture
- Seldom more than 5 cm in diameter except when due to overdosage with clomiphene or HMG (see p. 209)
- Often associated with:
  —anovulatory cycles
  —fertility drugs, as above
  —polycystic ovary syndrome (see p. 188)
- The majority are symptomless
- Pain (usually mild but sometimes severe) is due to rupture of or haemorrhage into the cyst. (If unilateral pain is accompanied by slight menstrual disturbance an ectopic pregnancy must be excluded.)

Management
- If ovarian enlargement estimated at 4–6 cm is found at pelvic examination, carry out pelvic ultrasound.
  —If the presumed diagnosis is a 'cystic ovary' rather than a neoplasm no immediate action is necessary
  —Re-examine in 2 weeks; a follicular cyst will usually have disappeared
  —If the cyst is unchanged or larger, further investigation (e.g. laparoscopy) is warranted.
- If discovered or confirmed by laparoscopy, the cysts can be aspirated. Laparotomy is not necessary.
- Send the fluid for cytology to definitely exclude neoplasia.
- Treat any underlying condition.

THECA-LUTEIN CYSTS

- A corpus luteum becomes cystic and persists in a functional state for longer than normal; or the granulosa and theca cells of a follicular cyst become luteinised.
- Characteristically, short periods of amenorrhoea are followed by heavier than usual uterine bleeding.
- The endometrium is secretory.
- (Haemorrhage from even a normal corpus luteum can mimic ectopic pregnancy closely.)

- Multiple and sometimes moderately large theca-lutein cysts are associated with trophoblast tumours. This is due to hCG stimulation.

Management
- Spontaneous resolution is usual.
- If a laparotomy is performed because of a mistaken diagnosis of ectopic pregnancy, interfere with the ovary as little as possible.

ENDOMETRIOTIC (CHOCOLATE) CYSTS

Due to ovarian endometriosis (see p. 199).

OVARIAN NEOPLASMS

- The incidence tends to rise with age but there is an increase in benign tumours in the fifth decade (40–49 years) and in malignant tumours from 50 years of age onwards.
- There is an association between ovarian cancer and:
  —nulliparity
  —social class (mortality in class I twice that in class V)
  —breast cancer—50% excess of ovarian cancer has been suggested if breast cancer is (or has been) present. This may be due to a genetic risk related to inheritance of the BRCA1 gene. Such families may account for 1–5% of ovarian cancer cases.
  —endometrial cancer—this relates mainly to endometrioid ovarian tumour and thecal cysts (see below).
- Oral contraceptives have the same protective effect as pregnancy. There may also be a protective effect associated with mumps virus.
- Ovarian tumours constitute 35% of all gynaecological malignancies. Although it is the sixth commonest in incidence, the ovary is the fourth commonest site for fatal malignant disease in the female, after breast, colon and lung.

HISTOLOGICAL TYPES AND DERIVATION

Three types of cells give rise to the vast majority of primary ovarian tumours:
- surface epithelium (mesothelium)
- germ cells
- gonadal stroma (sex cord stromal).

They may sometimes be mixed.

SURFACE EPITHELIAL TUMOURS

These tumours mimic tissues derived from the Müllerian or

paramesonephric duct. They comprise: serous papillary, mucinous, endometrioid and clear cell tumours, Brenner tumours and fibromas.

Serous papillary tumours

Benign: serous cystadenoma.

Malignant: serous cystadenocarcinoma.

- They account for about 10% of ovarian neoplasms, and are bilateral in about 50% of cases.
- Usually unilocular with a smooth outer surface. The internal papillae may sprout through the capsule giving an impression of malignancy. The lining cells are cuboidal or columnar, resembling the epithelium of the endosalpinx.

Mucinous tumours

Benign: mucinous cystadenoma.

Malignant: mucinous cystadenocarcinoma.

- They form 30–40% of ovarian neoplasms, and are often large, unilateral multilocular cysts.
- Loculi are lined by tall mucus-secreting columnar cells. They may be found along with a Brenner tumour (see below).
- Between 5 and 10% show areas of malignancy on removal.
- If the cyst ruptures, the mucus-secreting cells may implant on the peritoneum and produce the rare but chronic *pseudomyxoma peritonei*.

Endometrioid tumours

- These solid tumours frequently contain elements of both serous and mucinous tumours.
- There is a definite association with endometrial carcinoma, perhaps as a result of simultaneous neoplasia in tissue of common embryonic origin.

Clear cell ('mesonephroid') tumours

This may be a variant of the endometrial tumour because they often coexist.

Brenner tumour

- Unilateral and usually benign.
- Cords of squamous or transitional cells surround a central core lined by columnar epithelium. The fibrous tissue element closely resembles that found in a fibroma.

Fibroma

- Often moderately large, hard and lobulated with a glistening surface.

- Bilateral in about 10% of cases.
- The main interest of this rare tumour is its association with ascites and pleural effusion (usually right-sided) known as Meigs syndrome.

GERM CELL TUMOURS

Teratomas—arise from embryonic structures

Benign (mature tissues): dermoid cyst

Malignant (immature tissues): teratocarcinoma

- Dermoid cysts are the commonest ovarian tumours in young women.
- They are usually symptomless, but torsion or rupture may produce signs and symptoms of an acute abdomen.
- Bilateral in about 10% of cases and seldom larger than 12 cm in diameter.
- Lined by stratified squamous epithelium with its usual cutaneous elements—hair, sebaceous and sweat glands. Teeth, neural tissue, cartilage, alimentary and respiratory epithelium and even active thyroid tissue (*struma ovarii*) may be present.
- Solid teratomas may be benign but are usually malignant.
- The degree of malignancy and prognosis is related to the maturity of the component tissues.

True malignant change (usually squamous carcinoma) can develop in any of the tissue types found in a mature dermoid.

Extra-embryonic germ cell tumours

Choriocarcinoma and yolk sac (endodermal sinus) tumours

- These tumours produce pregnancy-associated plasma proteins, e.g.
  —choriocarcinoma: hCG (and human placental lactogen (hPL) to a lesser extent)
  —yolk sac: AFP.
- These can be used as tumour markers in diagnosis and follow-up after treatment.
- Malignant germ cell tumours have in the past had a bad prognosis. Intensive chemotherapy is now producing better results.

Disgerminoma

- A very rare tumour arising mostly between 20 and 30 years of age
- Arises from undifferentiated germ cells
- The counterpart of the seminoma in males
- Can usually be dealt with by conservative surgery, and is very radiosensitive. The preferred modern treatment is combination chemotherapy so that fertility can be preserved.

GONADAL STROMAL TUMOURS

- The stromal cells retain a potential for differentiation into any of the cells or tissues arising from the mesenchyme of the gonad (i.e. granulosa, theca, Leydig and Sertoli cells).
- These rare tumours may therefore secrete any or all of the ovarian steroids.
- They tend to be classified according to morphology:
  Granulosa – theca cell group which may produce oestrogen
  —Granulosa-cell tumour—not infrequently malignant but usually of low grade
  —Thecoma—fibroma

  Sertoli-Leydig cell group (which may secrete androgens)
  —Sertoli–Leydig cell tumour (androblastoma, arrhenoblastoma)
  —Sertoli-cell tumour
  —Leydig-cell tumour (hilus or lipoid cell tumour)

  Mixed—elements of granulosa cell tumour and arrhenoblastoma present (gynandroblastoma).
- Feminising (oestrogen-producing) tumours cause:
  —precocious puberty before the menarche
  —cystic glandular hyperplasia in menstruating women
  —postmenopausal bleeding in older women.

  There is an association with endometrial carcinoma.
- Masculinising (androgen-producing) tumours will initially result in defeminisation, including secondary amenorrhoea then hirsuties, enlargement of the clitoris and deepening of the voice.

SECONDARY OVARIAN TUMOURS

- Signs or symptoms referable to the breast, stomach, large bowel and uterus must be sought.
- The rare Krukenberg tumour usually results from simultaneous primary tumours in the gastrointestinal tract (particularly stomach) or breast and both ovaries.
- The histology is characterised by clumps of mucus-secreting epithelial cells in stroma. The mucin compresses the nuclei of each cell to one pole, producing 'signet-ring cells'.

CLINICAL FEATURES OF OVARIAN TUMOURS

- The peak age incidence is between 40 and 60 years, with the exception of teratomas and gonadal stromal tumours which occur at any age.
- Ovarian tumours rarely give rise to specific symptoms early in their course.
- The commonest presenting features are vague gastrointestinal upset (usually dyspepsia) or increasing abdominal girth, usually ascribed to 'middle age spread' by patients and medical attendants.

- This means that:
  —they are often found accidentally
  —if they are malignant the disease has commonly spread
   outside the ovary before the diagnosis is made.
- Abdominal swelling may be present but ignored by the patient.
- Menstrual function is not usually affected (except by the rare
  gonadal stromal tumours).

Differential diagnosis
Ovarian tumours must be distinguished from a whole variety of
pelvic and abdominal swellings. Among the most common are a
full bladder or rectum; corpus luteum; intrauterine pregnancy:
uterine fibroids; and hydrosalpinx.

Aids to diagnosis
- Ultrasound
- Laparoscopy
- Tumour markers—the results are, so far, disappointing except for
  the rare germ cell tumours.

CLINICAL FEATURES IN MALIGNANT VERSUS BENIGN TUMOURS

- *Age*—tumours in childhood are frequently malignant. In older
  women the risk of malignancy is proportional to age; 45% of
  tumours removed from women aged 45 years or over are
  malignant.
- *Pain and tenderness*—benign tumours are never painful unless
  complicated (see below). A sudden severe pain suggests torsion
  or rupture. Dull aching pain may suggest malignancy. Sacral
  nerve root pain is strongly suggestive of malignancy.
- *Rapidity of growth*—suggests malignancy.
- *Number of tumours*—75% of malignant tumours are bilateral,
  and 15% of benign tumours are bilateral.
- *Consistency of tumours*—solid, nodular and irregular growths
  are more likely to be malignant.
- *Fixation* is suggestive of malignancy, but not necessarily so.
- *Ascites* is usually a sign of peritoneal metastasis (especially if the
  fluid is bloodstained). Remember the possibility of Meigs
  syndrome (see above).
- *Oedema* of the legs and vulva or evidence of venous obstruction
  are suggestive of malignancy.
- *Metastatic deposits*. Remote metastases are not common, but in
  advanced disease supraclavicular nodes may become enlarged.
  The pouch of Douglas may contain irregular deposits which can
  be felt on bi-manual examination. *The majority of patients with
  ovarian cancer present with advanced disease.*

COMPLICATIONS OF OVARIAN CYSTS

- *Torsion.* Acute or subacute pain may be accompanied by mild shock. The lower abdomen is tender with guarding and rigidity. Pelvic examination reveals a tender adnexal mass. Laparotomy is indicated and removal of the ovary usually necessary.
- *Rupture.* The signs and symptoms will vary. The contents of chocolate (endometriotic) and dermoid cysts are extremely irritant and therefore may cause severe symptoms.
- *Haemorrhage* into or from cyst. The signs and symptoms will vary according to the degree of haemorrhage.
- *Infection.* This is not a common complication of ovarian tumours.
- *Malignant change.* This occurs mostly in serous and mucinous cystadenoma. New symptoms are not produced. It is commonly assumed that all malignant ovarian tumours develop from benign cysts; there is little evidence that this happens frequently.

Ovarian cancer screening
- Ovarian cancer kills about 4000 women per year in England and Wales.
- The population risk is 1:70 with a rise in incidence after 40 years of age.
  —Women with one affected relative may have some increase in lifetime risk
  —Two or more first- or second-degree relatives affected suggests a genetic predisposition (i.e. they may carry the BRCA1 or BRCA2 gene). Their lifetime risk of developing ovarian cancer may be up to 50%
  —Women in this group are also at more risk of breast, endometrial or colorectal cancer.
- The best available screening strategy combines vaginal examination, vaginal ultrasound (carried out by experienced personnel) and serum CA125 levels.
- There are problems with current screening methods:
  —Despite a relatively high sensitivity and specificity, the low prevalence of the disease means that the positive predictive value is only 10%; i.e. 10 women would require laparoscopy or laparotomy for every one cancer detected
  —Interval cancers occur as frequently as those detected; therefore screening would need to be carried out at least yearly
  —There is no evidence that screening reduces mortality, probably because it cannot detect the cancer early enough.
- On current evidence there is no justification for screening women at low or even moderate risk.
- Screening is probably justified in women with a strong family history (see above). Some opt for prophylactic oophorectomy with HRT around age 40 years.

- The protective effects of oral contraceptive use (see p. 221) should be borne in mind when counselling young women at high risk of ovarian cancer.

MANAGEMENT OF 'BENIGN' OVARIAN TUMOURS

- Laparotomy must be undertaken in the presence of any ovarian swelling >5 cm diameter, particularly if it is continuing to enlarge.
- A combination of the following features found at laparotomy may indicate (a higher risk of) malignancy:
  —the tumour is totally or partly solid
  —bilateral tumours
  —there is fungation through the capsule (not merely papillary growths)
  —large vessels on the tumour surface
  —blood-stained ascites
  —invasion of or adhesion to surrounding structures
  —metastatic deposits.
- If there is real doubt, a frozen section should be asked for.
- In tumours known or thought to be benign the treatment depends on the age and parity of the patient.
  —In young women who wish to conserve reproductive capacity, enucleation of the cyst (cystectomy) is carried out.
  —Larger cysts may demand removal of the ovary.
  —In women past child-bearing age it is customary to remove both ovaries and the uterus.
- If the cyst is unilateral, consider biopsy of the other ovary to exclude an occult tumour.

MANAGEMENT OF EARLY CARCINOMA OF THE OVARY

All the commoner malignant tumours are considered together because the stage and histological grading of the malignancy are more important prognostic indicators than the type of tumour.
- A midline or paramedian incision is required for full examination of the abdomen, particularly the diaphragm.
- *Accurate staging is vital*: see the information box.

Technique of staging
The following should be inspected and biopsied if involvement is likely or suspected:
- Peritoneal washings for cytology
- Parietal peritoneum
- Omentum
- Uterus and other ovary
- Bladder
- Pelvic peritoneum—biopsy if ovary is adherent
- Bowel and its mesentery
- Lymph nodes—para-aortic and pelvic; biopsy if possible
- Liver—surface and substance
- Diaphragm—both leaves.

Carcinoma of ovary: clinical staging	
Stage I:	Growth limited to the ovaries
Stage Ia:	Only one ovary involved; no ascites (sub-groups: capsule not ruptured; capsule ruptured)
Stage Ib:	Both ovaries involved; no ascites (sub-groups as above)
Stage Ic	One or both ovaries involved plus ascites or with malignant cells in peritoneal washing (sub-groups as above)
Stage IIa	Extension/metastases to uterus/tubes
Stage IIb:	Extension to other pelvic tissues
Stage IIc:	As IIa/b with ascites or positive peritoneal washing
Stage III:	Growth involving one or both ovaries with intraperitoneal metastasis
Stage IV:	Growth involving one or both ovaries with distant metastasis

Surgery (and adjuvant therapy?) in early disease

- The treatment of choice for stage I carcinoma of the ovary is bilateral salpingo-oophorectomy, hysterectomy and omentectomy.
- Simple oophorectomy may be indicated for younger women with stage Ia disease (and favourable histology) who wish to preserve their reproductive capacity and who fully understand the risks.
- Adjuvant therapy is not indicated for stage I disease unless:
  —the tumour is poorly differentiated
  —ascites was present
  —the cyst was ruptured.
- Single-agent chemotherapy is the preferred adjuvant but external beam radiotherapy may be used.

MANAGEMENT OF ADVANCED OVARIAN CARCINOMA

- Every attempt should be made to remove all macroscopic tumour.
- Single-agent chemotherapy is, in general, as effective as multiple-agent treatment.
  —An alkylating agent (such chlorambucil, melphelan or cyclophosphamide) or cisplatin/carboplatin can be used
  —Initial results using paclitaxel are encouraging.
- 80% of tumours respond to chemotherapy.
- Although complete remissions are possible, the long-term outlook with advanced disease is poor.

Survival rates for primary ovarian carcinoma

Stage Ia 85%; Stage Ib–IIa 40%; Stage IIb 25%; Stage IIc–III 15%; Stage IV <5%.

Second-look operations after 12 months?
- A policy of 'second-look operation', whether by laparotomy or laparoscopy, has not been shown to improve the survival of the patient.
- It may be justified with informed patient consent in chemotherapy trials.

Secondary 'debulking' operations
Patients who have chemotherapy to reduce the volume of cancer in the abdomen may benefit from a second operation to remove residual disease before further chemotherapy.

PAIN RELIEF IN ADVANCED MALIGNANT DISEASE

Definition
- Pain is an unpleasant sensation arising from stimulation of specific nerve endings, transmitted through more or less specific central nervous pathways to higher centres in the brain mainly located in areas which subserve emotion.
- Pain, emotion and personality are therefore inextricably linked.

PRINCIPLES

Aim to keep the patient both free of pain and fully alert.

Assessment
- Treatment varies according to the cause of the pain.
- The malignant disease may not be the cause of the pain.
- Some patients require a combination of drug and non-drug measures, e.g. radiation for bone pain, nerve blocks for nerve compression pain.

Choice of analgesics
- Establish a simple, practical analgesic 'league table', e.g.:
  —non-narcotic—aspirin (alternative paracetamol)
  —weak narcotic—codeine (alternative DHC, d-propoxyphene)
  —strong narcotic—morphine (alternative papaveretum, diamorphine).
- Analgesics should be given regularly to *prevent* pain: 'as required' medication is unacceptable.
- Doses should be determined on an individual basis; the correct dose is that which gives relief for at least 4 hours.
- Relief of pain should be assessed in relation to comfort achieved:
  —during the night
  —in the daytime at rest
  —on movement.

FURTHER READING

Burghardt E (ed) 1993 Surgical gynecological oncology. Thieme Medical Publications, Stuttgart

Coppleson M 1992 Gynecologic oncology, 2nd edn, Vol 2. Churchill Livingstone, Edinburgh

Shaw R W, Soutter W P, Stanton S L (eds) 1996 Gynaecology, 2nd edn. Churchill Livingstone, Edinburgh

Shepherd J J, Monaghan J M 1990 Clinical gynaecological oncology, 2nd edn. Blackwell Scientific, Oxford

Tindall V R 1990 Jeffcoate's principles of gynaecology, 5th edn. Butterworths, London

U K Co-ordinating Committee on Cancer Research 1989 Ovarian cancer screening.

26. The climacteric

- The *menopause* is the time at which menstruation ceases.
- The *climacteric* is the transitional period during which a woman's reproductive capacity ceases.
- The average age at which the menopause occurs is 51 years.
- A *premature menopause* is one which occurs before 45 years of age. It affects about 1% of women. Among the causes are:
  —genetic
  —metabolic
  —infection
  —auto-immune
  —iatrogenic—surgery, chemotherapy, radiation
  —idiopathic.

PHYSICAL CHANGES OCCURRING FROM THE MENOPAUSE

Ovaries
Cortical thinning occurs and the ovaries shrink in size (some hormone synthesis persists).

Genital tract
Changes in the vulva and vagina are gradual over many years:
- the labia shrink
- the skin of the vulva and vagina become atrophic
- the vagina becomes more smooth, narrower, less well lubricated and the pH rises
- the pelvic floor muscle becomes more lax with an increased risk of utero-vaginal prolapse.

The uterus is reduced in size:
- myometrial cells are partly replaced by fibrous tissue
- endometrium becomes atrophic.

Bladder and urethra
The epithelium thins and is more liable to infection.

Skin and breasts
- The epidermis and dermis become thinner and less elastic; sebaceous and sweat gland secretion decreases.
- The glandular tissue of the breast atrophies, being replaced by fat.

Cardiovascular systems
The levels of cholesterol, phospholipids and triglycerides rise. The risk of coronary artery disease gradually increases to the extent that it is the major cause of death in this group of women.

Skeleton
Calcium is lost from the bone at about 1% per year; gradual osteoporosis results.

SYMPTOMS ASSOCIATED WITH THE CLIMACTERIC

Symptoms frequently begin before the menopause. There are five groups of interlinked symptoms.
- *Vasomotor*—over 80% of menopausal women will have hot flushes and night sweats; the aetiology is not understood; it is not merely lack of oestrogen.
- *Emotional*—between 25 and 50% will complain of lethargy, lack of concentration, irritability, aggressiveness, depression, lability of mood, or anxiety.
- *Sexual*—decreased libido; dyspareunia—often due to atrophic vaginitis.
- *Urinary*, e.g. urgency and frequency of micturition—usually due to atrophic trigonitis and urethritis.
- *Musculo-skeletal*—laxity of ligaments and decreasing muscular strength may give rise to a variety of joint-related aches and pains.

Management
- General medical disorders (e.g. hyperthyroidism) need to be excluded.
- Therapy is of three main types:
  —hormones and other drugs
  —treatment of related disorders e.g. obesity, hypertension
  —psychological support.

HORMONE REPLACEMENT THERAPY (HRT)

- Cyclical oestrogen-progestogen therapy for women in whom the uterus is still present, *or*
- Unopposed continuous oestrogen orally or by implant, in women who have had hysterectomy.

ROLE OF HRT

- There is an increased risk of endometrial, and possibly breast, cancer when unopposed oestrogen replacement is given after the climacteric.
- If HRT is necessary in a patient who still has her uterus it should be given cyclically combined with progestogen for the last 7 to 13 days of the cycle.

- Outpatient endometrial sampling should be carried out if unopposed oestrogens have been taken for more than 6 months.
- Irregular vaginal bleeding is an indication for urgent biopsy or transvaginal scanning to measure endometrial thickness.
- There is no convincing evidence that HRT which includes progestogen per se increases the risk of breast cancer (see Further Reading).

CONTRAINDICATIONS TO HRT

Absolute
- Endometrial cancer
- Breast cancer
- Undiagnosed vaginal bleeding
- Undiagnosed breast lump
- Suspected pregnancy
- Severe active liver disease.

Relative
- Hypertension
- Past history of thromboembolism
- Diabetes mellitus
- Gallstones
- Uterine fibroids
- Endometrial hyperplasia
- Otosclerosis
- Migraine
- Malignant melanoma
- Benign breast disease.

Other drugs for vasomotor symptoms
- Clonidine improves vasomotor symptoms for some patients.
- Propranolol does not reduce hot flushes but may help tachycardia or palpitations.
- Psychotropic drugs are not appropriate for purely menopausal symptoms.

Duration of treatment
This depends on the informed choice of each woman. The balance of benefit is probably towards continuation for as long as possible.

POSTMENOPAUSAL BLEEDING (PMB)

All cases must be thoroughly investigated (except perhaps for the withdrawal bleeding which occurs at the expected time in menopausal women taking HRT). Investigations must include:
- complete pelvic examination
- cervical smear
- endometrial biopsy—this can often be achieved as an outpatient. If not, proceed to hysteroscopy and directed biopsy.

FURTHER READING

Rees M (ed) 1995 Menopause update. Postgraduate series. Reed Healthcare Communications, London
RCOG 1996 Postmenopausal women: HRT today and into the future. British Journal of Obstetrics & Gynaecology 103:Suppl. 13
Studd J W W, Whitehead M I (eds) 1988 The menopause. Blackwell Scientific, Oxford

27. Gynaecological surgery

PRE-OPERATIVE ASSESSMENT

- The correct operation must be carried out for the correct reasons. If the management suggested in outpatients is found not to be appropriate at the time of admission it must be altered accordingly or deferred for further investigation as appropriate.
- Women who smoke and are scheduled to have a general anaesthetic should be advised to stop smoking several weeks before the proposed operation.
- For women on the combined pill see page 223
  —Advice about alternative contraception must be given.
- Outpatient assessment must include:
  —general physical examination, including breasts, cardiac and respiratory status and BP
  —haemoglobin and blood group estimation
  —ECG and chest X-ray, urea and electrolyte estimation in hypertensive women.
- Anaemia should be corrected before admission.
- Among the patients who require particularly careful assessment are:
  —those with medical disorders such as cardiac disease, hypertension, diabetes mellitus or other endocrine disorders
  —those on treatment which may affect their response to anaesthesia or surgery, e.g. antihypertensives (particularly β-blocking agents); psycho-active drugs (particularly mono-amine oxidase inhibitors); anticoagulants; systemic corticosteroids
  —the morbidly obese (e.g. BMI >39/m^2); this is a significant risk factor in post-operative morbidity and mortality.
- Blood should be sent in good time to allow grouping and saving of serum or cross-matching depending on the extent of the surgery involved.

PRE-OPERATIVE SELECTION

DAY-CASE SURGERY

- Each unit must have *pre-operative selection guidelines* for day-case surgery such as the following:

—The patient should be fit and healthy or, at most, have *mild* systemic disturbance from the condition to be treated or other pathology

—Any patient taking long-term medication must be carefully assessed and discussed with the anaesthetist

—Patients who are morbidly obese, have imperfectly controlled diabetes mellitus, chronic respiratory or cardiovascular disease are *not* suitable for day-case treatment

—Although all patients should be judged on physiological rather than chronological age, treatment of a woman >60 years as a day case needs to be considered carefully

—Day-case treatment is inappropriate if the proposed surgery has a significant risk of causing severe post-operative pain and/or haemorrhage

—If general anaesthesia is to be used (or may be required), no solid food should be taken for 6 hours or clear fluid for 3 hours pre-operatively

—The operation should not normally exceed 60 minutes' duration.

- The patient should be seen by the surgeon before discharge when an explanation of the surgery can be given.
  —She should not be discharged until she is fully recovered, awake and with stable vital signs.
  —Control of nausea and pain must be adequate.
  —She must be accompanied home by a responsible adult.

MINIMAL ACCESS GYNAECOLOGICAL SURGERY (MAGS)

ADVANTAGES/DISADVANTAGES

Among the *suggested benefits* are:
- less post-operative pain
- shorter hospital stay
- more rapid recovery
- fewer wound-related complications
- lower incidence of post-operative respiratory complications and ileus.

Disadvantages include:
- increased operation time
- greater risk of iatrogenic complications (related to experience of the surgeon).

PRINCIPLES

- MAGS and 'day-case' surgery are not synonymous. Full pre-operative assessment is required—'short-cuts' must be avoided.
- MAGS requires some different skills compared with open surgery. These must be learned and the 'learning curve' varies among individual surgeons.

—All surgeons still have to be skilled at 'traditional' operative techniques before embarking on MAGS procedures
—An experienced colleague must supervise the initial cases of a surgeon undertaking a technique new to him or her ('proctoring')
—*Some gynaecological surgeons may not have the aptitude to perform MAGS safely and effectively.*
- MAGS involves risk that must not be underestimated.
- Those carrying out MAGS must adhere to basic surgical principles of open procedures, e.g. it requires meticulous haemostasis.
- Surgical specimens should be available to the pathologist for diagnosis, particularly if malignant disease is suspected.

LAPAROSCOPIC SURGERY

Stratification of laparoscopic procedures by levels of training
- The RCOG has produced the following guidelines for training in laparoscopy and hysteroscopy (see Further Reading).
- It does not mean that all procedures listed have been shown to be superior and more safe than their 'open' alternatives. *Better designed trials are required especially for the more advanced techniques.*

Level 1—Diagnostic laparoscopy

Level 2—Minor laparoscopic procedures
- Laparoscopic sterilisation
- Needle aspiration of simple cysts
- Ovarian biopsy
- Division of minor adhesions (not involving bowel)
- Diathermy to mild endometriosis.

Level 3—More extensive procedures requiring additional training
- Laser/diathermy to polycystic ovaries
- Laser/diathermy to moderate endometriosis (including endometrioma)
- Salpingostomy
- Salpingectomy/salpingo-oophorectomy
- Ovarian cystectomy
- Laparasocopically assisted vaginal/sub-total hysterectomy
- Division of moderate/severe adhesions (including bowel involvement).

Level 4—Extensive endoscopic procedures requiring subspecialist or advanced/tertiary level skills
- Myomectomy

- Laparoscopic surgery for major endometriosis
- Pelvic lymphadenectomy
- Pelvic side wall/ureteric dissection
- Dissection of an obliterated pouch of Douglas
- Laparoscopic procedures for incontinence.

- For Levels 1–3 the trainee's performance should be supervised by a trained endoscopist until confirmed competent.
- Level 4 procedures are the province of those nationally/internationally recognised in the field of MAGS.

COMPLICATIONS OF LAPAROSCOPIC SURGERY

The non-lethal complication rate is reported to be about 1/1000 for diagnostic laparosocopy and 5/1000 for more advanced procedures. These figures can be related to:
- mode of access in which the Verres needle or trocars may damage abdominal wall or major intra-abdominal blood vessels, bowel or bladder
- performance of the operation—particularly risk of damage to ureter, bladder, rectum or pelvic blood vessels
- anaesthetic problems, e.g. due to production of a CO_2 pneumo-peritoneum or prolonged maintenance of lithotomy position.

HYSTEROSCOPIC SURGERY

The basic principles of hysteroscopy are different from laparoscopy and must be learned separately.

Stratification of hysteroscopic procedures by levels of training

Level 1—Diagnostic procedures
- Diagnostic hysteroscopy
- Removal of simple polyps
- Removal of IUD.

Level 2—Minor operative procedures
- Proximal fallopian tube cannulation
- Minor Asherman's syndrome
- Removal of pedunculated fibroid or large polyp.

Level 3—More complex procedures requiring additional training
- Division/resection of uterine septum
- Major Asherman's syndrome
- Endometrial resection/ablation
- Resection of submucous fibroid.

COMPLICATIONS OF HYSTEROSCOPIC SURGERY

Intra-operative	Early post-operative	Late post-operative
Uterine perforation	Infection	Recurrence of
Intra-abdominal	Secondary	symptoms
injury	haemorrhage	Pregnancy
Fluid overload	Haematometra	(Uterine malignancy)
Haemorrhage	Cyclical pain	
Gas embolism	Treatment failure	

PERIOPERATIVE COMPLICATIONS

The National Confidential Enquiry into Perioperative Deaths (NCEPOD) in the UK (see Further Reading) makes it clear that, where major or minimal-access surgery is carried out:

- essential services such as recovery rooms, high dependency and intensive therapy units must be ready and available
- proper equipment and qualified specialist staff must be available at all times
- any surgeon or anaesthetist must be competent to deal with the immediate hazards which may occur during an operation, such as haemorrhage or cardiac failure.

THROMBOEMBOLISM (TE)

- Deep vein thrombosis (DVT) and TE are important perioperative complications in gynaecological surgery. DVT is detected in about 12% of women undergoing abdominal hysterectomy. It is likely that many go undetected in all types of surgery.
- TE is associated with 20% of perioperative deaths after hysterectomy.
- In the majority of patients dying from pulmonary embolism the preceding thrombosis had not been detected.

Risk markers for TE

These are listed in the information box.

Patient-associated factors	Disease/procedure-associated factors
• Increasing age • Obesity • Severe varicose veins • Immobility (bed rest >4 days) or paralysis • Pregnancy or puerperium • Previous TE • 'Thrombophilia'*	• Abdomino-pelvic surgery • Malignancy, especially pelvic, abdominal, metastatic—accounts for 35% of cases • Infection • Polycythaemia, paraproteinaemia, paroxysmal nocturnal haemoglobinuria • Nephrotic syndrome • Inflammatory bowel disease • Cardiac failure or recent MI

*e.g. deficiency of protein C, protein S, or antithrombin III; activated protein C resistance; anti-phospholipid syndrome and lupus inhibitor

Prophylaxis against TE

Prophylaxis reduces the risk of fatal and non-fatal TE. Methods are listed in the box below.

Prophylaxis against TE	
Mechanical methods	e.g. graduated elastic compression stockings or intermittent pneumatic compression
Pharmacological methods	Low-dose subcutaneous heparin will prevent 60–70% of DVTs and fatal PE; low m.w. heparins may be more effective in high risk patients.
caution required with spinal/epidural anaesthesia	Warfarin • can be given as perioperative low dose (1 mg daily) but this needs further evaluation, or • at full dose postoperatively in high risk patients; keep INR[1] at 2.0–2.5. Dextran 70—not so effective in preventing DVT. Anti-platelet agents (e.g. aspirin) of limited efficacy?

[1] INR—International Normalised Ratio of the prothrombin time

Contraindications to heparin include:
- hepatic or renal failure
- peptic ulcer or oesophageal varices
- previous hypersensitivity to heparin
- severe hypertension
- thrombocytopenia
- von Willebrand's disease.

THRIFT and the RCOG (see Further Reading) suggest the following guidelines for prophylaxis.
- **Low risk**—*early mobilisation and hydration required*
  —Minor surgery (<30 min); no other risk markers
  —Major surgery (>30 min); age <40 years and no other risk markers.
- **Moderate risk**—*consider one of a variety of prophylactic measures available*
  —Minor surgery (<30 min) in women with a personal or family history of TE or thrombophilia
  —Major surgery (>30 min)
  —Extended laparoscopic surgery
  —Obesity (>80 kg or BMI >30/m²)
  —Severe varicose veins
  —Current infection
  —Immobility for >4 days before surgery
  —Major current illness (see risk markers above)
- **High risk**—*Use heparin prophylaxis (with leg stockings)*
  —A total of three or more moderate risk markers above
  —Major abdominal or pelvic surgery for malignant disease
  —Major surgery (>30 min) in women with a personal or family history of TE or thrombophilia *or* paralysis or immobilisation of lower limbs.

Management of suspected or established thromboembolism
- The symptoms and signs of pulmonary embolism (PE) can be missed.
- Typically there is pleuritic pain, haemoptysis, dyspnoea and various degrees of hypotension.
- It may, however, present with dry cough, pyrexia, tachycardia or bronchospasm. There may or may not be evidence of a preceding DVT.
- Collapse and sudden death can occur.
- The differential diagnosis includes chest infection, pneumothorax, aspiration, and myocardial infarction.

Investigation
- Arrange venography for DVT and a ventilation perfusion isotope lung scan if PE is suspected.
- Chest X-ray; ECG; and blood gases may help to identify other causes.
- If TE is confirmed screen for thrombophilia—if present seek advice of haematologist.

Treatment
- The aim is to prevent extension of existing thrombus and prevent further complications.
- Acute treatment is with calcium heparin intravenously for at least 48 hours.

- Warfarin should be commenced and continued for at least 3 months. The correct dosage maintains the INR at 2.0–2.5.

Surgery and the COC pill—see page 223.

Surgery and HRT
There is no increased risk of TE (in the absence of other risk markers).

VAULT-HAEMATOMA AND PELVIC INFECTION

To prevent this, the following are recommended:
- pre-operative vaginal preparation with povidone-iodine
- complete haemostasis during surgery
- adequate drainage of the pelvis
- prophylactic broad spectrum antibiotics for abdominal and vaginal hysterectomy.

WOUND HAEMATOMA AND DEHISCENCE

- A transverse suprapubic incision should be used when possible but is not appropriate for management of ovarian cancer.
- Aseptic technique is vital.
- Haemostasis and closure techniques are important.
- A non-absorbable or polyglycolic acid suture is preferred for closure of the rectus sheath.
- Drainage must be adequate.
- The risk is increased slightly if low-dose heparin is being used as prophylaxis against TE.

URINARY TRACT COMPLICATIONS

- The incidence of *urinary infection* can be reduced by eliminating catheterisation as much as possible.
  —The patient is asked to void urine before the premedication is given. A distended bladder can be emptied during the operation by syringe and needle if needs be.
  —If continuous bladder drainage is necessary postoperatively a suprapubic catheter should be used.
- *Injuries* to the urinary tract are preventable, but if they occur prompt recognition at the time and appropriate remedial action are required. If an injury is not detected for some time after surgery it should await tissue healing and elimination of infection before repair is attempted.

FURTHER READING

Campling E A, Devlin H B, Hoile R W, Lunn J N 1995 The Report of the National Confidential Enquiry into Perioperative Deaths 1992/1993

Morris P, Malt R A 1995 Oxford textbook of surgery, Vols 1, 2. Oxford University Press, Oxford

RCOG 1994 Training in gynaecological endoscopic surgery. RCOG, London

RCOG Working Party on Prophylaxis against Thromboembolism in Gynaecology and Obstetrics 1995: Report. RCOG, London

Sutton C (ed) 1993 New surgical techniques in gynaecology. Parthenon Publishing Group, Carnforth

Sutton C, Diamond M (eds) 1993 Endoscopic surgery for gynaecologists. Saunders, London

THRIFT Consensus Group 1992 Risk of and prophylaxis for venous thromboembolism in hospital patients. British Medical Journal 305:567–574

Index